PRIDE OF AMERICA
WE'RE WITH YOU

Pride of America
We're With You

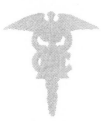

The Letters of Grace Anderson

U.S. Army Nurse Corps, World War I

SHARI LYNN WIGLE

SEABOARD PRESS

AMERICAN VOICES SERIES, J. A. ROCK & CO., PUBLISHERS

Pride of America, We're With You: The Letters of Grace Anderson,
U.S. Army Nurse Corps, World War I by Shari Lynn Wigle

SEABOARD PRESS

is an imprint of James A. Rock & Company, Publishers

THE AMERICAN VOICES SERIES
Memoirs of America's Living Past

Pride of America, We're With You: The Letters of Grace Anderson,
U.S. Army Nurse Corps, World War I copyright © 2007 by Shari Lynn Wigle

Special contents of this edition copyright ©2007
by Seaboard Press

Front Cover Photos:
Dressing Station, Ambulance Co. No. 316 (see Chapter 4, photo 28)
Camp Pike nurse group (see Chapter 2, photo 16)
Grace Anderson at Camp Pike (see Chapter 2, photo 18)
Back Cover Photos:
Grace Anderson in Army Nurse Corps Uniform (see Chapter 3, photo 22)
Army Nurse Corps Insignia 1907-1920

Address comments and inquiries to:
SEABOARD PRESS
9710 Traville Gateway Drive, #305
Rockville, MD 20850
E-mail:
jrock@rockpublishing.com   lrock@rockpublishing.com
Internet URL: www.rockpublishing.com

Trade Paperback
ISBN: 978-1-59663-772-6

Library of Congress Control Number: 2006935793

Printed in the United States of America
First Edition: 2007

To Ellen, Grace, Martha Rose, and Dana,

the four generations who saved

the World War I memorabilia

for ninety years and made

this book possible.

To Erik and Anna, the fifth generation —

May you appreciate and remember the

sacrifices and contributions of

your great-grandparents and

all Americans who served

in the Great War.

Acknowledgments

Lynn Swan, my niece, invited me to read the rediscovered World War I letters and presented me with an intriguing writing and research opportunity. She and her husband, Dana Swan, entrusted me with the story of his grandmother, Grace Anderson. Dana, the fourth generation to save Grace's Great War collection, supported the project at every level. Lynn, who envisioned the book, organized and managed the memorabilia. She offered inspiration and ideas from the first skeletal version to the final one.

Toni Bronson, my sister, listened to my daily reports of progress and challenges, continually encouraged me, and shared valuable feedback on all the drafts. My late parents, Jack and Helen Wigle, contributed by shaping my thinking and enabling my education and career goals. Ron Bronson, my brother-in-law, helped the computer-related technical aspects go smoothly. Erik and Anna Swan, Grace's great-grandchildren, cheered me on and so did my nephews, Randy, Ric, and Rob Bronson, and their families.

Kathy McLendon, who has a software engineering background, assisted with proofreading, another talent of hers. Anne Ruck, Marianne and Lyle Reeves, all teachers, motivated me with their enthusiasm for the book. Lyle gave me insights, based on his American history expertise. Lianne Ericsson, the daughter of a World War I veteran and a registered nurse, advised me on nursing terminology.

Jim and Lynne Rock introduced me to book publishing and answered this neophyte's numerous questions. With their thirty-five years of publishing experience, they guided me through the process of turning my manuscript into a James A. Rock & Company, Publishers title. John T. Greenwood, PhD, Chief, Office of Medical History, Office of the Surgeon General, U.S. Army, reviewed parts of chapters and provided U.S. Army photos, illustrations, and insignia from World War I. Sharon Schroeder, librarian-archivist, Goodhue County Historical Society in Red Wing, Minnesota, found key information on Red Wing and the Anderson family.

Table of Contents

Photo Credits

Several photos in this book are used with permission from the Office of Medical History, Office of the Surgeon General, U.S. Army. The photos are identified with their figure numbers from the army history book, a brief description, and the chapter location in *Pride of America, We're With You,* in the order of appearance. All photos depict medical facilities in France except Figures 90 and 91 which, as noted in the list, are from Germany.

The following photos are from *The Medical Department of the United States Army in the World War*, Volume 2, *Administration American Expeditionary Forces.*

131   Base Hospital No. 17, Dijon, *Chapter 4*
120   Ward, Base Hospital No. 1, Vichy Hospital Center, *Chapter 5*
97   Surgical ward, Allerey Hospital Center, *Chapter 6*

The following photos are from *The Medical Department of the United States Army in the World War*, Volume 8, *Field Operations*. All appear in *Chapter 4.*

59   First Aid Station, 1st Division, back of front-line trenches, Missy-aux-Bois
61   Dressing station entrance, Ambulance Co. No. 111, 28th Division, near St. Gilles
69   Wounded walking to dressing station, Argonne Forest
87   Dressing Station, Ambulance Co. No. 316, 79th Division, Les Eparges, Meuse (also on the front cover)
50   Church at Bezu-Le-Guery used as ward by Field Hospital No. 1, 2nd Division
56   Triage, 42nd Division, located near Suippes
14   Adjusting improved splint on a litter patient, Broussey
60   Field hospitals of the 4th Division at Chateau de la Foret
51   Evacuating wounded by truck, Field Hospital No. 15 near Montreuil

Other photos from Volume 8, *Field Operations,* are:

9   Hospital train, method of loading, *Chapter 5*
90   American Hospital and Infirmary, Neuenahr, Germany, *Chapter 7*
91   Surgical and medical wards, American hospital group, Coblenz, Germany, *Chapter 7*

Other U.S. Army images appearing in *Pride of America, We're With You* are:

Army Nurse Corps Insignia 1907–1920 from the Army Nurse Corps Historical Collection, Office of Medical History

France in 1918 Map from the *United States Army in the World War*, Volume 1. Washington: U.S. Army Center of Military History, 1988

Army Forces in Germany map from the Research Collections, Office of Medical History

Photo of Veteran Affairs, Los Angeles National Cemetery by Shari Lynn Wigle

All other photos in *Pride of America, We're With You* are used with permission from the Anderson Wells Memorabilia, a private collection.

List of Photos

The photo numbers and the abbreviated captions are in the order of appearance in *Pride of America, We're With You*.

Introduction

When we get ready to sail everything will be very quiet. We will leave our quarters without any luggage and when we are on board, our boat will slip away some night [1] ... We nurses are provided with rubber suits, which keep one afloat and warm & dry for forty-eight hours ... These suits are complete even to rubber caps & whistles around our necks so we can call for help ...[2]

In 1918 Grace Matilda Anderson of the U.S. Army Nurse Corps described the secrecy of her New York embarkation and the Red Cross survival gear for German submarine attacks in the Atlantic. Why did Grace and thousands of other nurses trade their jobs and the safety of United States soil for World War I overseas duty?

Grace and the nurses of Base Hospital Unit No. 115 answered that question in their song.

We'll soon be with you boys,
To share your joys, your sorrow, pain and everything.
We're glad you're there, we're glad that we are coming, too,
To help you to win the victory.
Pride of America, we're with you,
All of our strength we'll gladly give you ...[3]

The stirring lyrics reappear here and in their entirety in chapter three. Nearly ninety years ago the Base No. 115 nurses gathered in New York to sing of their devotion to America and her armed forces. The melody and the chorus of one hundred women from every corner of the country are long forgotten. Yet their heartfelt words recapture the harmony of their thoughts and actions.

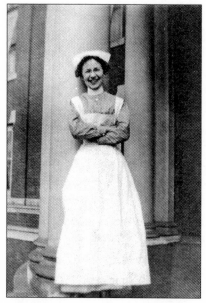

Grace Anderson studied nursing from 1913 to 1916 at Northwestern Hospital, Minneapolis. (1)

Patriotism, self-sacrificing spirit, and dedication to their profession motivated Grace and more than ten thousand other U.S. Army nurses[4] to volunteer for a perilous venture. Those grandmothers of baby boomers offered their medical expertise without adequate pay, rank or benefits. They crossed the Atlantic to aid troops, who fought to preserve democracy, before American women gained the right to vote.

Grace joined the corps unaware of how the Great War, which affected millions of people in myriad ways, would reach into her mind and heart. She contributed a year and a half of her life to a massive montage of personal experiences produced by the war.

As a nurse anesthetist, Grace helped save soldiers in operating rooms and wards. She healed "our boys" and her own heartaches – a life-changing romance and the tragic loss of a loved one. Grace's story, based on her letters from 1917 to 1925, follows her during the U.S. transition from neutrality to involvement in the war, and from training at Camp Pike, mobilization in New York, nursing assignments in France and occupied Germany, to the postwar period and afterward.

In her correspondence Grace praised her patients for their bravery in the hospital and on the battlefield. She loved caring for them but felt the pain of their plight. "I would be very happy here if I didn't have so much heartache for these boys of ours ... Their spirit is wonderful. But to see so many cripples and mutilations ..."[5]

Grace thought that writing about her wartime responsibilities would worry her parents. So she gave them many glimpses of her activities outside the hospitals. Grace told about the fascinating but frigid living quarters in a Dijon palace and a Vichy hotel. She endured icy cold bath water and scolded the steam radiator with "a kick or a knock"[6] every time she got near it.

Berths on an American train in France pleas-

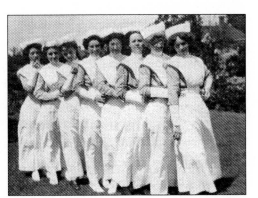

Grace, second from right, and her friends took a break from their nursing school classes to line up for this picture. (2)

antly surprised Grace as did "a real breakfast on a diner"[7] in contrast to feeling "packed in like sardines … without being able to lie down"[8] on previous trips. In Vichy she witnessed "people shouting, everybody wildly happy"[9] at an armistice celebration. In occupied Germany she saw "Germans stop and take off their hats to our flag."[10]

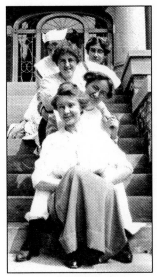

Grace, second from bottom, and her classmates had fun posing for the camera on the steps of Northwestern Hospital. (3)

Dana Swan, who remembers his grandmother's World War I anecdotes, saved her memorabilia for several years. Dana and his wife, Lynn, almost lost the collection in January 2005 when they converted an office-storage room into a walk-in pantry. During a flurry of cleaning and remodeling, cardboard boxes holding the letters and photos mistakenly landed in a discard pile. Lynn spotted an envelope postmarked 1918 and rescued the Great War treasure, kept by four generations, before it became trash.

Because of a home improvement project and serendipity, the Swans rediscovered the mementos that withstood household moves across the country and within California. Lynn believed Grace's story should be shared beyond their children, Erik and Anna, and their descendants. Her vision inspired this book.

Military censoring or personal reasons prevented Grace from sending all her news. She promised to tell everything when she returned. The undisclosed information included her romance with Capt. George Dillard Wells, a U.S. Army Medical Corps officer. The narrative relates that intriguing and complicated aspect of her life. Dates and duty stations in their military records re-created the timeline of their relationship.

The narrative also interweaves Grace's correspondence with World War I history, the U.S. Army base hospital system, U.S. Army Nurse Corps, and details of people, places, and events she mentioned. Her slang, abbreviated sentences, use of the ampersand, words such as "till" and "tho," and names of most family members and relatives remain.

Grace, born in Red Wing, Minnesota, in 1884, was among hundreds of thousands of Americans who went to the Great War as first or second-generation immigrants. Her father and her paternal and maternal grandparents were natives of Norway.

Grace's father, Andreas Fredrick Andersen, emigrated from Norway to America at age twelve with his parents and his four siblings. In the United States Andersen family members eventually changed the spelling of their name to Anderson. In a biography Fredrick recounted their journey that started in his namesake birthplace.

We started from Fredrickshald for America on the 5th day of May 1857, and we went through Hamburg in Germany … Then we came on a sailing ship called Diana to New York. They used no steamers in those days and we were eleven weeks on the ocean. We arrived in New York the last part of August 1857.

The journey across the Atlantic was quite rough. Father, for purpose of safety, concealed his gold money in a leather belt around his waist from which he suffered a great discomfort, as it chafed and lacerated his flesh. We left New York by rail to Chicago, Illinois, and from Chicago by railroad to Davenport, Iowa. We took a steamer called the War Eagle up the Mississippi River, and came to St. Paul the first part of September 1857.[11]

Fredrick and his family settled near St. Paul where they cleared timber, built a house, and farmed the land. Fredrick began military service at age fifteen with the Home Guards "out against the Indians until the spring of 1862."[12]

Ellen Matilda Wilson, Grace's mother, also experienced adventures at age fifteen. In 1862 Ellen and her family traveled via oxen team from Wisconsin to Red Wing, through unsettled territory. They chose a different route when riders warned them of an Indian uprising and massacre. Along the way the Wilsons assisted farmers in a small community harvest crops because most of their men were fighting with the Union army in the Civil War.[13]

Fredrick married Ellen in 1870 and bought an eighty-acre farm, where they resided for four years. The Andersons moved to Red Wing and raised eight children, two of whom died at young ages. The citizens of Goodhue County elected Fredrick sheriff four times from 1886 to 1895. An owner of hardware and general merchandise stores, Fredrick also engaged in business interests such as farmlands, banking, and manufacturing.[14]

Grace, the Andersons' youngest daughter, learned about catastrophic events at age six, long before World War I. Her teenage brother, Arthur,

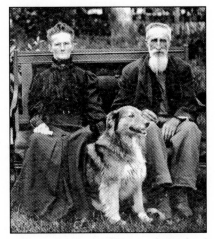

Grace's parents, Ellen and Fredrick Anderson, shown here with the family dog at their home in Red Wing, Minnesota, were married in 1870 and raised eight children.(4)

survived one of the deadliest river disasters to occur on the upper Mississippi.[15] During an evening storm in July 1890, the steamboat *Sea Wing* capsized. Most of the ninety-eight passengers who perished were Red Wing residents.[16]

In 1906 Grace and her parents celebrated her father's retirement by taking a six-month trip to Europe. They visited Norway and Sweden, the Andersons' native countries, as well as England, France, and Germany. Grace, an alumna of Red Wing High School, graduated from Northwestern Hospital Association Training School in Minneapolis as a registered nurse in 1916. She worked at Northwestern Hospital and completed an anesthetist course before joining the army.

Grace followed two of her brothers into the medical field. Fredrick Edward practiced dentistry in Red Wing for more than six decades. Clarence, a physician and surgeon, served on the Mayo Clinic staff at the same time as Dr. William J. Mayo and Dr. Charles H. Mayo, the founding brothers.

When Grace left Minnesota for Camp Pike and the war, the Anderson family had lived in Red Wing for over forty years. Three generations of Andersons, highly respected citizens, helped lay the foundation and build the community.

In the tradition of her parents and grandparents, Grace possessed the same hardy pioneer spirit. So did other nurses who journeyed "over there" to support the troops in the struggle for liberty. As the ninetieth anniversary of the November 11, 1918, armistice approaches in 2008, we salute Grace and the American nurses of World War I. The actions of all mirrored the poignant pledge of the Unit No. 115 song: "Pride of America, we're with you – All of our strength we'll gladly give you …"[17]

CHAPTER 1

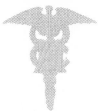

Answering
America's Call

*"I am very glad to go … I haven't the least fear or worry
in the world. Am ready for anything."*[1]
—Grace Anderson

The United States involvement in World War I ignited a patriotic fervor for country and cause that swept from coast to coast. At train stations bands played and crowds waved flags as their boys headed for training camps. Rousing rallies boosted sales for Liberty Bonds. To save wheat and meat for the army, loyal adults and children ate fish and planted vegetable gardens. Nurses signed up for duty near the battlefront and at behind-the-lines hospitals.

Grace Matilda Anderson enthusiastically volunteered as an army nurse in November 1917. In contrast, after the war broke out in August 1914, Grace preferred following the conflict from Minnesota because she agreed with the U.S. policy of neutrality. Grace, a nursing student whose family had ties to Europe, sympathized with the suffering victims. She understood why civilians responded when both the Allies and Central powers requested American assistance.[2]

In September 1914 nurses and doctors sailed from New York to France on the SS *Red Cross*, a mercy ship, to aid combat wounded, regardless of allegiance. Hundreds of altruistic men and women

1

crossed the Atlantic to help both sides at foreign hospitals, welfare and relief agencies. At home several organizations sustained the afflicted abroad.[2]

Grace, like the majority of U.S. citizens, eventually directed her compassion to the Allies exclusively as a result of Germany's hostile actions. A German submarine torpedoed the British steamship *Lusitania* and killed over one hundred Americans and more than one thousand other civilians. After Germany promised to stop unrestricted submarine warfare, U-boats sunk cargo vessels of the United States and other neutral and friendly nations. The British intercepted and decoded the Zimmermann Telegram and sent it to the U.S. government. Americans' anger intensified when the deciphered message revealed a German plot to entice Mexico to invade its northern neighbor.[3]

President Woodrow Wilson called for war against Germany, which Congress declared on April 6, 1917. Most people zealously applauded the declaration of war and thousands of men proudly joined the armed forces. Opponents objected to getting involved and having a large standing army and conscription. Wilson faced the challenge of quickly moving the populace through a transition from neutrality to full support of the war efforts.[3]

The country, completely unprepared for battle, needed to raise an army of millions. Wilson, who realized an all-volunteer army could not amass the enormous military force required for victory, proposed a "selective" draft system. In May 1917, Congress passed the Selective Service Act, which established 4,648 local draft boards.[4]

Wilson and the government formed a Committee on Public Information to motivate all Americans to adopt his battle cry, "the world must be made safe for democracy." He appointed George Creel, an investigative journalist, as chairman. Creel pleaded the justice of America's cause to unite the minds and hearts of the one hundred million population in passionate determination.[5]

Creel, influential and controversial, attracted thousands of volunteers including prominent artists, scholars, writers, historians, and speakers for CPI branches throughout the nation. Long before global mass media and advanced technology, Creel and his staff communicated innovatively using the written and spoken word, telegraph, cable, and wireless. The CPI created synergism with pamphlets, posters, advertising, news releases, syndicated features, speeches, motion pictures, still photos, stereopticon slides, and exhibits at state fairs and war expositions.[5]

Grace worked at Northwestern Hospital in Minneapolis as a registered nurse after the U.S. entry in the hostilities. She typified what her fellow citizens experienced during the rapid transformation. She read CPI pamphlets explaining America's ideals and aims and saw CPI advertising, donated as free space, on billboards, in newspapers, and magazines.[5]

Grace listened to some of the Four Minute Men, a group of 75,000 speakers in 5,200 communities. She attended four-minute talks in Minneapolis and Red Wing, where the orators were friends of her father, Fredrick Anderson. The Four Minute Men energized audiences with 755,190 war-related speeches. They appeared at civic events and any available public gathering at military camps, schools, churches, and especially movie theaters, where silent film stars attracted crowds of fans.[5]

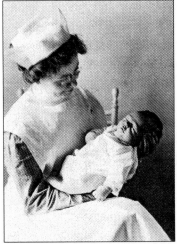

Grace enjoyed taking care of her youngest patients at Northwestern Hospital in Minneapolis. (5)

Captivating visuals and persuasive slogans of full-color posters reinforced the spirited spoken messages. The CPI tapped into the power of the popular lithographs, dominant mass communicators in the years before television and national radio. The United States printed twenty million posters, more than all the other belligerent nations combined, during its nineteen months in the war.[5]

The impressive art touched the lives of Grace and everybody across the country. Inexpensive posters, dis-

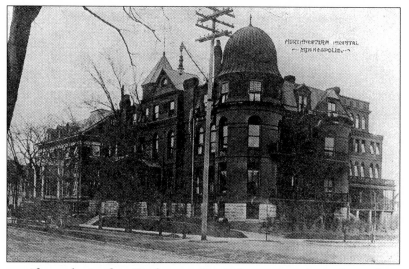

After graduating from Northwestern Hospital as a registered nurse in 1916,
Grace joined the hospital's nursing staff. (6)

played in banks, stores, schools, hospitals, and post offices, played a
starring role in the CPI campaign. Placards rallied participation in
the U.S. government's World War I goals and programs, based on
the theme of making a just and lasting peace.[5]

Everywhere young men looked Uncle Sam pointed directly at
them and proclaimed: *I Want You for the U. S. Army.* James Mont-
gomery Flagg illustrated the enduring image. Over four million
copies of the classic poster were printed in 1917 and 1918. *Gee!! I
Wish I Were a Man, I'd Join the Navy* by Howard Chandler Christy
depicted a charming woman posing in a sailor suit. She enticed
thousands of young men to navy recruiting stations. Some armed
forces recruits, fired up by promotional imagery, lied about their
age so they could go to France and defeat the Germans.[5,6]

The first draft turned into an impassioned nationwide festival
in spite of some opposition to Selective Service. Boat horns, whistles,
and church bells announced the start of registration. Civic, political,
and military leaders delivered lively speeches about duty and the country's
needs. Attendees marched in loyalty parades to the drumbeat of bands
and sang optimistic Great War era songs like "Over There."[6]

With the stirring tunes ringing in their ears, about ten million men between the ages of twenty-one and thirty-one registered on June 5, 1917. The next year registration reached nearly twenty-four million after two more drafts and a new age range of eighteen to forty-five.[6]

Beginning with fewer than 130,000 pre-war regular soldiers, the War Department mobilized 4,734,991 draftees and volunteers for World War I. Over 500 men represented Red Wing, Grace's small hometown, in every branch of service. A total of 4,057,101 served in the army and air service; 599,051 in the navy, and 78,839 in the marines. The troops who voyaged to France numbered 2,086,000.[6]

To ensure that immigrants would fight for their new country, the government introduced "100% Americanism." The expression signified absolute loyalty to the United States and its wartime goals. Almost half a million foreign-born men, drafted into the army, arrived in America between 1880 and 1920 as part of a massive influx of over twenty-three million immigrants. The U.S. armed forces also included thousands of the foreign born who enlisted prior to the draft and thousands of second-generation immigrants.[7]

For *Americans All!* Howard Chandler Christy portrayed a patriotic woman placing a wreath on an honor roll of fourteen ethnic names. "100% Americanism" caught on across the nation. Since Grace's father and her paternal and maternal grandparents emigrated from Europe, the phrase resonated with the Andersons.[7]

Grace and her family accepted Wilson's challenge to prove they were "100% American" by purchasing war bonds. The hoopla of marching bands and speakers launched four Liberty Loan campaigns and one Victory Loan drive. All economic levels of the populace could afford the bonds, offered in all denominations. The U.S. government expected everyone from laborers to millionaires to take ownership of the war effort by personally financing it. States, counties, and cities staged sales rallies to achieve their bond quotas suggested by the federal government.[7]

Five hundred thousand copies of *That Liberty Shall Not Perish from the Earth*, by Joseph Pennell, implored the public to invest in

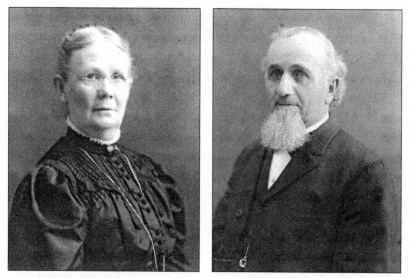

Grace's parents, Ellen and Fredrick Anderson, second and first-generation immigrants, respectively, supported "100% Americanism." (7 & 8)

Liberty Bonds. Few could resist when they saw the stark picture of the Statue of Liberty, with her head floating in the ocean, and New York under a blazing attack by airplanes and ships.[7]

The Liberty Bond publicity reaped big rewards. The contributions of Grace, her family, and over 8,600 residents of Red Wing helped their Goodhue County exceed its $6,080,000 quota by $225,000. Many generous communities surpassed their quotas. As a result, the federal government raised $23 billion from a population with a total annual income of less than $70 billion.[7]

As a member of the War Savings Stamps committee, Grace's father persuaded his relatives and the townspeople to buy stamps so they could assist the troops and earn interest. *Joan of Arc Saved France* by Haskell Coffin featured a dramatic Joan of Arc holding her sword high and beseeching: "Women of America, Save Your Country - Buy War Savings Stamps." Even school children used their piggy bank coins for the stamps that sold rapidly in Red Wing and elsewhere. Anderson and the committee brought in more than $300,000, nearly half the savings stamps sales of Goodhue County.[7]

The food conservation program and its catchphrase, "Food Will Win the War," focused on women because they cooked the meals. Drawings of fish, poultry, and grains or baskets of colorful vegetables and fruits coaxed everybody to eat those foods. Adults and children cultivated home and school gardens. Families conserved for the soldiers by consuming less sugar and fats and observing "wheatless" and "meatless" days.[7]

The Committee on Public Information's successful publicity also caused some problems. To foster America's fear of the enemy, the government presented Germans as villains and exaggerated their evil actions in pamphlets, posters, and speeches. Consequently, people feared the German language, books, and even threatened German Americans. The CPI then tried to redirect anti-German sentiment to the real enemy in Europe. Fortunately, the good side of patriotism prevailed. So did the country's generosity that extended beyond Liberty Bonds and War Savings Stamps to several civilian organizations.[8]

Many posters sought volunteers and solicited donations for the American Red Cross. For *10,000,000 Members by Christmas,* C. B. Falls drew a holiday candle illuminating a large red cross in a window. The message was "On Christmas eve a candle in every window and Red Cross members in every home." For *Hold Up Your End!,* William B. King showed a Red Cross nurse lifting one end of an army cot.[9]

The Andersons and other families put candles in their windows and held up their end of the cot so the Red Cross could sponsor extensive projects at home and abroad. From 1914 to 1918, the membership soared from about seventeen thousand to almost thirty-two million adults and juniors. In 1918 there were over eight million volunteer workers and the public contributed $400 million in money and materials.[9]

The Red Cross continuously enlisted more nurses, one of its most important missions. An abundance of illustrations highlighting nurses in capes and caps or hospital uniforms circulated throughout the nation. Women responded to the emotional appeals like

"They Need Us Over There," and "Nurses of America, Humanity Calls You. What is Your Answer?" "Help!" expressed the thoughts of a nurse trying to carry an injured soldier.[10]

The Red Cross endeavor to enroll nurses to aid the servicemen tugged at Grace's heart. In November 1917 she decided to leave her Minneapolis hospital job. She wanted to care for the sick and wounded troops in France.

Grace became one of the twenty-nine thousand nurses the Red Cross recruited for its own ranks, the army, navy, and public health service at home and overseas.[10] In 1901 the female U.S. Army Nurse Corps was established as an acknowledgment of the value of women nurses in modern war. During World War I the ANC expanded from four hundred to more than twenty-one thousand.[11]

Grace's belief in the justice of the cause and her hope for ultimate peace in the world inspired her. She knew the Great War would be costly in financial and human terms but she planned to "do her bit," in the "war to end all wars."

Another factor influenced Grace's decision. She fit the profile of the American "new woman," who emerged and developed in the late nineteenth and early twentieth centuries. She was single, self-reliant, middle class, and well educated. Although devoted to her parents, her siblings, and her hometown, she also welcomed living independently in a city.[12]

As a new woman, Grace moved outside the domestic realm and into the public sphere. She admired her civic-minded father, elected county sheriff four times. She acquired his interest in local, national, and world issues and enjoyed discussing current events. Grace utilized her innate nurturing abilities and her desire to serve humanity in community pursuits and one of the professions chosen by new women – teaching, nursing, and social work.[12]

Major cultural changes such as urbanization and industrialization provided Grace and other women opportunities to broaden their horizons and embark on unfamiliar adventures. During World War I women entered the workforce and fought harder for equal rights. The consciousness-raising suffrage movement strengthened women, who were close to obtaining the right to vote nationally.[12]

The National Woman's Party emphasized the irony of the United States fighting in the Great War to preserve democracy and at the same time denying women suffrage. When the NWP picketed the White House, the police arrested and jailed the activists who went on a hunger strike. Wilson freed the suffragists and they resumed protesting.[12]

Grace approved the approach of the National American Woman Suffrage Association. The NAWSA participated in the full gamut of war activities and toiled in hospitals and factories on the home front. They counted on their patriotism to gain Wilson's support for their cause.[12]

Spurred on by wartime idealism, Grace told her parents: "I am very glad to go and whatever happens, everything is all right. I haven't the least fear or worry in the world. Am ready for anything."[13]

On October 2, 1917, less than two months before Grace joined the army, a noteworthy event occurred in the U.S. Army Nurse Corps. Gen. John J. Pershing, commander in chief of the American Expeditionary Forces, cabled a request to the War Department for "a competent member of the Nurse Corps" to supervise nursing in the AEF. Bessie S. Bell, chief nurse of Walter Reed General Hospital, reported for duty on November 13, 1917.[14]

Two weeks later on November 27, 1917 the Army Nurse Corps of the War Department, Office of the Surgeon General, Washington, D.C., issued these orders.

"With the approval of the Secretary of War, Grace M. Anderson of Minneapolis, Minnesota – Reserve Nurse, Army Nurse Corps, is hereby assigned to active service in the military establishment, and will enter upon her duties after taking the oath prescribed by Section 1757 of the Revised Statutes of the United States ... Oath of Office taken December 1, 1917 in the County of Hennepin, Minnesota."[15]

At the Red Wing train station, as Grace bid goodbye to her family, the shrill whistle and the "all aboard" signaled the first leg of

ARMY NURSE CORPS

WAR DEPARTMENT
OFFICE OF THE SURGEON GENERAL
WASHINGTON

NOVEMBER 27th, 19 17.

With the approval of the Secretary of War,

GRACE M. ANDERSON

of　　MINNEAPOLIS,　　MINNESOTA,

Reserve Nurse, Army Nurse Corps, is hereby assigned to active service in the military establishment, and will enter upon her duties after taking the oath prescribed by Section 1757 of the Revised Statutes of the United States.

Bertw. Caldwell
Major, Medical Reserve Corps.
For the *Surgeon General, U. S. Army.*

Oath of office taken
December 1, 1917, in the
County of Hennepin, Minnesota,
before
Filed in S.G.O.,

Bertlis Caldwell
Major, M.R.C., U.S.Army.
W.D., S.G.O., December 7, 1917.

*The U.S. Army Nurse Corps assigned Grace to active service
on November 27, 1917. (9)*

her journey to World War I. She realized her second trip to Europe
would transcend her previous pleasure excursion. In 1906 Grace
and her parents traveled by rail to New York and by steamer across
the Atlantic for six months of sightseeing. News from "over there"
warned her about the risks, uncertainty, and danger but to no avail.
She heard a summons more powerful than the familiar shout of the
train conductor. America called Grace and she answered.

CHAPTER 2

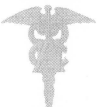

Waking
to the Bugle

There are a fine lot of men here. Our army ought to
make a smash when they get over there.[1]
—Grace Anderson

Grace journeyed by rail from Red Wing and her civilian life to Little Rock and an astonishing new realm, a World War I army cantonment. Amazed at seeing thousands of trainees at Camp Pike, Grace wrote: "No one seems to know how many men there are here, but there are men and men & men[2] ... The road outside here is full of soldiers marching just as far as I can see."[3]

Before Grace arrived at the camp nearly twenty-two thousand volunteers and draftees started basic training. The recruits, mainly from Arkansas, Alabama, Mississippi, and Louisiana, drilled, used rifles, and moved in small military units.[4]

Men traveled to sixteen National Army cantonments, each with space for thirty to fifty thousand troops. The National Guard filled another sixteen camps. The army named the installations, across America, for distinguished U.S. soldiers. Camp Pike honored Gen. Zebulon Pike, a nineteenth century western explorer, who discovered but never climbed the 14,110-foot Pikes Peak in Colorado.[4]

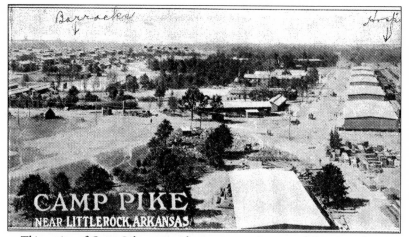

This section of Camp Pike appeared on a panoramic postcard Grace sent home.
She noted "barracks" and "hospital" at the top. (10)

The Camp Pike site, on the heights overlooking Little Rock, encompassed fifteen thousand acres. The government selected central Arkansas for its sufficient labor, materials, railroad connections, abundant water, and adequate drainage. The construction of cantonments presented monumental challenges.[4]

The War Department, which eventually raised and mobilized an army of more than four million, required multiple installations to house, train, and deploy troops to Europe. The department set a ninety-day deadline for building thirty-two camps, which began in the summer of 1917, the same time as the first draft.[4]

In July thousands of laborers, carpenters, plumbers, and electricians swarmed over the Arkansas property to transform timber, pastures, and farms into a cantonment. They turned most of the bucolic acreage, a haven for crops and cattle, into a mock battlefield for military maneuvers. Workmen constructed about three thousand structures for barracks, warehouses, hospitals, and stables for thousands of horses and mules.[4]

The colossal project consumed thirty million feet of lumber, seventy thousand windows, and ten thousand doors. Crews brought two railroad lines to the installation, where hundreds of miles of roads linked facilities. The army called up thousands of men quickly and increased the numbers monthly, creating a larger national military force than originally planned. The government's changes kept builders at Little Rock and at other locations toiling beyond the deadline.[4]

In September recruits streamed into an unfinished camp. Grace also noted construction activity when she reported for duty five months after the workers tackled their daunting tasks.

Camp Pike - Dec. 4, '17

Dear Mother,

Just a line to let you know I have arrived. The trip down was pleasant and I had some nice company. Had three hours in St. Louis but spent most of it in the station.

They are certainly nice to me here, so far it seems very pleasant & interesting. I cannot say how big this cantonment is – no one seems to know how many men there are here, but there are men and men & men. The camp is four miles across to the hospital, and they are building on the other side of the hospital. They say when it is finished the hospital will be in the center. That will make the camp eight miles long.

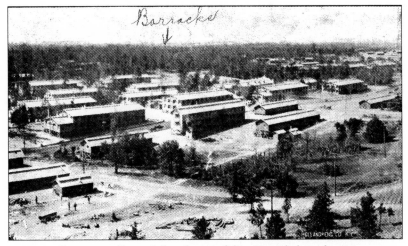

Grace wrote "barracks" at the top of this postcard photo showing another part of Camp Pike. (11)

There have been three thousand patients in the hospital but as near as I can make out there are between one & two thousand now. It is going to be some life down here. It is very warm here today. Too warm to wear a coat. Things are fairly convenient – steam heat, electric lights & bathrooms. Much love to you & Papa, Grace

Camp Pike - Dec. 9, '17
Dear Mamma,

Will you please send my wool quilt to me, and if you have a blanket to spare send me that too. The weather turned suddenly cold, and while it is beautiful outdoors, we feel the cold at night. These army blankets are heavy and stiff and somehow do not keep out the cold. Have longed for my little wooly quilt several times.

I think I will like it here soon as I get a little more used to it. We have fine meals. You needn't tell people how we fare, because they might think we fared too well. I'll tell you tho. For breakfast we always have fresh fruit of some kind, cereal, eggs & bacon or maybe steak and french fried potatoes, pancakes & syrup, toast and coffee. Lunch – soup, mashed potatoes & meat of some kind, two vegetables, salad, bread & butter & cake or cookies or custard or something like that. Dinner – potatoes, some other kind of meat, a couple of vegetables, salad, olives or pickles, and pie (usually).

And the cooking is excellent. Just like home cooking, even the bread, cookies, tarts & pies. I eat like a horse because I'm in the air a good deal. I'm so sorry for the poor boys in the army. They don't have a very easy time. Had my picture taken today in Red Cross cape & cap. Will send one home when I get them.

Dec. 10 –

You know if people lived in these buildings in Minnesota they would freeze to death. There is no foundation – the buildings are set up on posts, the outside boarded up and inside the walls are covered with a heavy sort of paste-board. The water pipes froze for us a day or so ago but have been thawed out now.

Just got your letter. It's the first letter I've had. You know I don't get homesick very easily because I've been out so much but this week I've had a few little twangs.

The nurses are very nice and am getting used to it but my, we have lots of awfully sick men. Have worked with both white men and Negroes down here. Lots of well educated young chaps are just common soldiers and it is hard on boys who are used to good things to be in with the rough element. I hope Joe [her sister, Josephine] will see that Sonny [Joe's son] is put somewhere he can be trained so he can be an officer if he must go to war, and you can't tell but what he will have to in time.

I wrote a letter for one of the common soldiers a day or so ago asking some friends to help him get into an officers' training camp. He has pneumonia but is getting better. I could tell by his language and his appearance that he is from a good family and it goes against him to rough it. Was so sorry for him. And there are lots of others.

Tell Papa that flashlight is going to come in fine. On night duty the nurses say the corridors are just pitch dark. Am glad he thought of it because I never did. We are very crowded and roughing it, but are well and fairly comfortable.

The road outside here is full of soldiers marching just as far as I can see. It is funny to wake in the morning hearing a bugle call, and to go walking out here and suddenly have a soldier with a gun cry "Halt!"

Army life is not easy. It is surely one of self-sacrifice. Sunday and Monday are just the same here, as far as our work goes, as we have to be on duty just as long.

The nurses' new quarters will soon be ready and we'll be snug as can be. In the mean time I'm borrowing one of the night nurse's bedding to add to mine and am warm enough at night till mine comes. Perhaps I'll have to send my laundry home. They only do our uniforms here. Much love, Grace

World War I army nurses usually worked in cantonment hospitals prior to their lengthy voyage across the Atlantic. During the camp period the army assessed the health, stamina, and professional capability of the women. While being evaluated, they adapted to military nursing before facing combat duty.[5]

As Grace transitioned to army life, she found pleasant surprises - steam heat, electric lights, bathrooms, and delicious food. She liked the unexpected home-cooked meals because, as a civilian, she adhered to "wheatless" and "meatless" days. Grace ate fish and vegetables to save for the troops, unaware that she would be in the army some day.

Grace also encountered unforeseen twists and turns along the way. She traded her comforts of home for roughing it. The nurses endured inadequate laundries, lack of bedding, working seven days a week, and "pitch dark" corridors connecting the main structure to additional buildings and wards. They adjusted to their surroundings, as Grace did, by sending laundry home or borrowing missing items.

In December 1917 one thousand to two thousand patients, according to Grace's estimate, occupied the hospital, which previously treated as many as three thousand. The soldiers became ill with pneumonia, as she mentioned. Measles, mumps, and meningitis also spread in a series of epidemics through the crowded camps.[5]

Grace's comment about her patients being "both white men and Negroes down here" reflected the racial prejudice in America in 1917. Although African-Americans served the United States honorably in previous wars, discrimination against them continued. Whites considered blacks as second-class citizens and also second-class soldiers.[6]

The army segregated the blacks, some of whom were sons of former slaves, in separate regiments. Mostly prohibited from fighting in battle, blacks labored behind the lines. They performed sanitary duty, unloaded ships, loaded trains and trucks, dug trenches, and buried soldiers killed in action. The few black units that engaged in battles fought bravely and helped win the victory.[6]

During the war 13 percent of U.S. Army personnel were black. At that time blacks composed only 10 percent of the American population. More whites than blacks staffed draft boards, which granted more deferments to whites. Selective Service drafted one in three blacks compared to one in four whites.[6]

The "well educated young chaps" put in with the "rough element" troubled Grace. Because of the unique demographic pattern in World War I, most trainees experienced some kind of culture shock at cantonments. Men left their jobs at farms, factories, and in various trades from blacksmiths to motor vehicle mechanics. Some claimed American colonists as ancestors and others had sailed to New York and lined up with the masses at Ellis Island.[6]

Only 21 percent of the drafted enlisted men had education beyond grammar school. Many of the country boys, 52 percent of recruits, saw motion pictures or attended lectures and concerts for the first time. The illiterates, 37 percent, could not read books or write letters like everybody else. The half million immigrants, who could not speak, read or write in English, and the second-generation immigrants made up 39 percent.[6]

To address training, socializing, and educating the recruits, Secretary of War Newton D. Baker created the Commission on Training Camp Activities. Social welfare agencies and ethnic leaders assisted the CTCA at special schools. Teachers, chaplains, and bilingual immigrants instructed the illiterates and the foreign born. The mandatory classes ensured that all the men could communicate with one another and understand military orders.[7]

Trainees learned basic reading, writing, and key military terms such as drill, tent, rifle, shoot, march, and bayonet. Instructors, who taught English with the universal language of pictures, used copies of *National Geographic Magazine* to make textbooks. The men studied English three hours a day, usually for four months.[7]

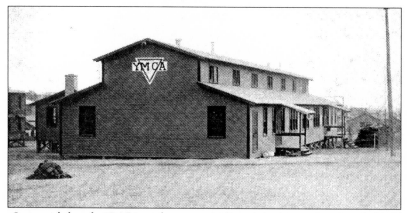

Grace said that the YMCA at the camp was "certainly doing a lot of work for the Boys." One auditorium held four thousand men.(12)

The army respected the Old World culture of foreign-born soldiers, who represented forty-six different nationalities. While guiding them through an Americanization process, the military encouraged immigrants to take pride in America as well as in their native country. The foreign born became better acquainted with the United States through classes in civics and citizenship. At the same time they enjoyed ethnic heritage events, homeland songs, and library books and newspapers in several languages. Many immigrants became U.S. citizens at hundreds of naturalization ceremonies held at army camps.[7]

In addition to their schooling, immigrants and illiterates participated in sixteen weeks of training with other soldiers. For forty hours per week they practiced military combat skills including trench and open warfare, signaling, hand grenade throwing, scouting, patrolling, and target shooting.[7]

Camp Pike - Dec. 15, '17
(A postcard showing a panoramic photo of the camp)
Everything fine down here, including weather. Getting more interesting all the time. Am feeling fine and gaining in weight, I'm sure because I eat so much. The only drawback is the distance from town.

This does not show all of the cantonment. The YMCA is certainly doing a lot of work for the Boys. They have two or three buildings here. One auditorium holds 4000. The Knights of Columbus also have a building. Write soon.

Much love, Grace

The YMCA, Knights of Columbus, YWCA, Jewish Welfare Board, Salvation Army, American Library Association, and other organizations supported the CTCA social, recreational, and educational activities. The social welfare staff steered troops away from alcohol, gambling, and prostitution. They directed recruits to wholesome pursuits to boost their morale and keep them physically and mentally healthy. The CTCA music festivals, plays by touring companies, bands, and choirs exposed lower class trainees to middle class culture.[7]

The YMCA's buildings and "work for the Boys" impressed Grace. In auditoriums, which seated two to four thousand, the YMCA and CTCA sponsored lectures, religious services, community singing, theater productions, weekly motion picture shows, and celebrations. The YMCA published a weekly newspaper of events for all the camps and provided the amenities of home such as pianos, books, phonographs, and stationery.[7]

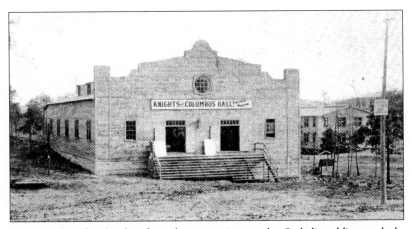

The Knights of Columbus focused its attention on the Catholic soldiers and also welcomed everyone, regardless of race or religion, to the clubhouse for recreation. (13)

The YWCA hostess houses or huts, designed with cafeterias, sitting rooms, verandas, and children's nurseries, bustled with activity on visiting days. Female workers staffed the homey and respectable places where soldiers socialized with women and relatives. The American Library Association sent nearly three million books and thousands of periodicals to libraries at all the installations.[7]

The Knights of Columbus and the Jewish Welfare Board planned religious services for Catholic and Jewish men. Many were immigrants from southern and eastern Europe. The two organizations eased cultural and religious challenges of the military, dominated by Anglo Saxon Protestants prior to World War I. The Knights of Columbus primarily looked after Catholics, an estimated 35 percent of the troops. However, they welcomed everybody, regardless of race or religion, to their clubhouses to watch motion pictures or use sports equipment, player pianos, and phonographs.[7]

In France Salvation Army huts attracted battle-weary Americans, who lined up for popular homemade donuts, distributed with cheerfulness and concern. The Salvationists, recognized for their overseas work, also brought their famous donuts, concerts, and song services to the cantonments.[7]

Camp Pike - Jan. 9, '18
Dear Mother,

Am beginning to like army life very very much and if it was not for the lack of hot bath water and clean clothes to wear, I should be very happy here. We hear a great deal of talk about overseas, but I don't think we'll be going for sometime.

As usual, I'm writing to ask for something. It is a shame to have to bother you, but I've been asked to teach anesthetics and must have my notebook. I think it is with my other nursing books in the bottom of my trunk. It is very warm here – hope I don't have to stay all summer. Am having a good time and am feeling fine. Hope everyone is well at home. My love to all, Grace

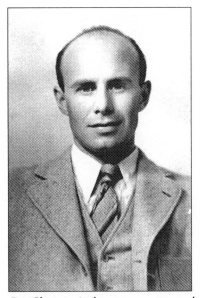

Dr. Clarence Anderson, a surgeon and Grace's brother, helped train her as a nurse anesthetist.(14)

Although Grace joined the army as a regular nurse, Medical Corps officers at Camp Pike soon noticed her expertise in anesthetics. When asked to teach anesthesia administration, Grace got in on the ground floor of a new program. The U.S. military trained nurse anesthetists for the first time during World War I. As early as the Civil War, nurses gave anesthetics to patients, while being supervised by surgeons, but without official military instruction.[8]

Grace earned her assignment because of her previous hospital experience in anesthesia, which she attributed to her brother, Clarence, a surgeon. Grace and Clarence, the two youngest Anderson children, formed a close bond that continued into adulthood. Grace admired her brother's achievements as a doctor and decided to enter the medical field.

After Grace graduated as a registered nurse, Clarence suggested that she study nurse anesthesia administration, which had been evolving since the late nineteenth century. Surgeons in the late 1800s faced a major concern, the high morbidity and mortality resulting from anesthesia. Some surgeons, especially William J. and Charles H. Mayo, thought nurses could solve the anesthesia problems. The Mayos believed intelligent nurses, with proper instruction, could become competent anesthetists who would concentrate fully on patient comfort and safety.[8]

The notebook that Grace hoped her mother would send contained the post-graduate course, given by Clarence and his colleagues, and her Mayo Clinic information. When Clarence became the assistant physician-surgeon in the section of roentgenology (the study

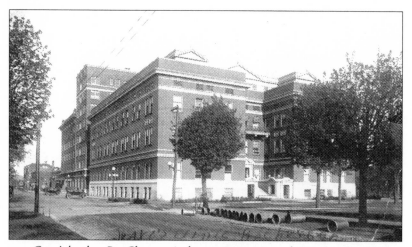

Grace's brother, Dr. Clarence Anderson, was assistant physician-surgeon in the roentgenology department at Mayo Clinic. (15)

and use of X-rays) at Mayo Clinic, he arranged for Grace to observe the techniques of highly skilled nurse anesthetists. Medical personnel from the United States and throughout the world traveled to Rochester, Minnesota, to learn from the Mayo brothers and their staff, renowned in surgery and anesthesia.[8]

Through her studies, observation, and hospital duty, Grace developed technical proficiency in open-drop ether administration. The method involved pouring ether from a special bottle that dropped the anesthetic onto a gauze-covered mask. After inhaling the fumes, the patient went to sleep.[8]

Grace belonged to a small group of army nurses who, before U.S. entry in the war, learned how to administer anesthesia. The women received their training from surgeons, on-the-job in hospitals, and from the first schools and educational programs for nurse anesthetists, which began in 1909. The army sought anesthetists and recommended the training to other nurses so they could expand beyond their usual responsibilities. As a result, Medical Corps surgeons acquired a valued resource, nurse anesthetists, in wartime operating rooms.[8]

Camp Pike - Jan. 25, '18

Dear Mother,

Thank you so much for my laundry. It is so nice to get really clean clothes. The laundries here are so short of fuel that they only run part of the time. We have not had clean uniforms for three weeks.

Am in the officers' ward now and having a good time. Nobody very sick and they are so good to us. Am getting rested up. Army life is getting very interesting and am glad I'm here.

We hear rumors of our going overseas soon & of our leaving for Greece. Ten of our nurses will go but do not know yet who. Next time you send me anything please put my nice night gowns & a boudoir cap and that blue silk bed jacket in the package. You will find them at the top of my trunk. Much love & will write again soon, Grace

Camp Pike - Jan. 26, '18

Dear Mother,

Am well and happy and anxious for the next step – foreign service. We may not get it but nearly all of us want it. There are a fine lot of men here. Our army ought to make a great smash when they get over there.

Will send you a picture of the hospital the same time I mail this. Hope you are not worrying about me. This place is doing me lots of good. Tell papa I have taken out $10,000 insurance. The income will go half to papa and half to you if anything happens to me. Oceans of love to you and Papa and the rest, Grace

Grace and almost all members of the armed forces, including army and navy nurses, purchased war risk insurance policies, mostly for the $10,000 maximum. The government managed the World War I insurance and deducted low rates monthly from the pay of the insured. After the war, policies could be converted to other life policies or an endowment.[9]

Camp Pike - Feb. 22, '18

Dear Mamma,

Have a little cold and am off duty for awhile. My room-mate was sick this week. Don't worry as I'm all right only they don't want to run any risks so they put me to bed.

Have gained four pounds so you can see I've been well and am in good condition. Oceans of love to you all. Like the work better all the time. Grace

Camp Pike - Feb. 25, '18

Dear Mamma & Papa,

After getting your letter I was afraid you would be worried by hearing that I'm under the weather a little. But have only been feeling bad a week and only in bed five days. Fever is leaving and there is no indication of any serious trouble. Feel good enough to get up today. A nurse from Red Wing arrived here today, Lorana Teele. Was glad to see her. Will write more soon. Much love, Grace

Camp Pike - Mar. 7, '18

Dear Mamma & Papa,

Received the box and many thanks for the clothes & also for the "eats." That was certainly nice of you, and tasted delicious. There is to be a very grand review here one of these days for Gen. Sturgis and I have an automobile at my disposal for that time, so expect to see it. The car belongs to one of the officers (a fine man), and is a beauty, so expect a good time.

Took a walk to the trenches yesterday. We also went down into the dugouts, underground rooms, thirty or more feet below the surface of the ground. The French officers here tell us the climate & conditions here are about the same as in France and from what I read, I guess it is so. There is water in the trenches all the time, and even in the dugouts, tho in the dugouts it is more mud. They will have floors in the dugouts after awhile.

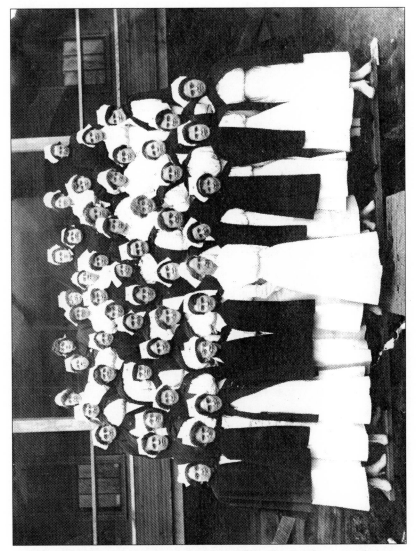

Grace (second row from bottom, third from left) and nurses from several states trained at Camp Pike. This photo is also on the front cover. (16)

It is like summer here now when the sun is shining, but gets a little chilly on dark days. Everyone but me is wearing summer or spring suits and straw hats. Write when you have time. Oceans of love, Grace

Camp Pike - Mar. 18, '18
Dear Mamma & Papa,

Shall finish my term of night duty now. Have four wards to look after and there are about two hundred patients. We were in the woods & picked violets today. Peach trees & all fruit trees have been blooming for some time.

We had a big Review here last Monday for General Sturgis who has just returned from France. It certainly was a sight to see those thousands upon thousands of men marching, and all the paraphernalia of war. It makes you realize there really is a war.

Hope the cold weather lets up pretty soon up there, and that you have a nice spring. A Canadian was telling me yesterday that the snow is nine feet deep in Canada.

How are Fred [her brother] and Nell [Fred's wife] and children & Arthur [her brother] & family. Give them all my

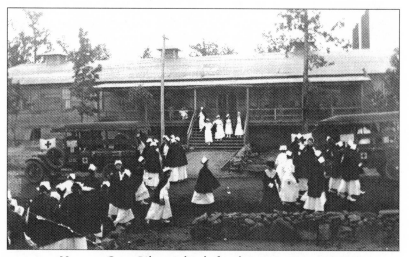

Nurses at Camp Pike socialized after their group picture. (17)

love. Please send me Floyd's
[her brother] address next time
you write.

Love to you all, Grace

Camp Pike greeted Maj. Gen.
Samuel Davis Sturgis Jr. with a big
review because he commanded the
Eighty-seventh Division, which
organized at the Little Rock installation. Before the Eighty-seventh
Division left Arkansas in June
1918, the men prepared for the
battlefields at trenches in the man-
euver area.[10,11] French officers, veterans of the front lines in France,
showed trainees how to attack and
defend a trench line and protect
themselves against poison gas.[11]

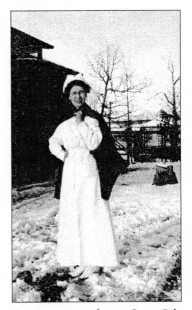

*A snowy winter day at Camp Pike
reminded Grace of her home state.
This photo is also shown on the front
cover. (18)*

Camp Pike - Mar. 29, '18
Dear Mamma & Papa,

Am almost thru with my night duty and am feeling fine.
There isn't much to write about today, just a line to let you
know I'm well. Life here is busy as ever but like it better all the
time. Hope you are all right, and that it is getting warm again.
Our weather is still fine. Much love to all, Grace

For two months Grace heard rumors about going overseas. The
American Expeditionary Forces continually lacked the required
number of nurses. Only two thousand had sailed to Europe by March
31, 1918. Two weeks later an acute shortage of more than one thousand nurses and other medical department personnel threatened a
breakdown in service to soldiers. An AEF cable on May 3 requested
that over five hundred nurses be transported immediately.[12]

The top priority of troops in the shipping schedule and not enough vessels resulted in the AEF's insufficient number of nurses. At times as many as 1,400 waited in the New York mobilization station to get space on ships. Although the AEF desperately needed the Camp Pike nurses, they remained in Arkansas until transportation improved. At the same time, the army required the services of thousands of nurses in the United States. During 1918 soldiers at all U.S. camps averaged over 1.3 million monthly.[12]

Camp Pike - May 16, '18
Dear Mamma,

Many thanks for sending my uniforms so promptly. I am getting along fine, riding horseback, playing volleyball, and soon our tennis court will be done. So you see we are having some good times as well as lots of work.

This hospital has twenty five hundred beds now. Hard to realize isn't it. It is a big place. I thought about you last Sunday, "Mother's Day." We had nice services in our chapel. Secretary of War Baker's wife was here last week. She is a very fine woman. She came to see the Operating Rooms and I was introduced to her. She is very unassuming in her manner.

Have my insurance papers arrived at home yet? The weather here has been perfect lately. Arkansas can be very attractive. Don't know when we go overseas but we may be called anytime. If you get a telegram saying – "Will be with you in spirit," you will know I'm sailing. But don't worry, as I'll surely have time to write you a letter before leaving this Camp. Am glad the hardest work came when I first came down here. It gets easier for me all the time now. I'm practically my own boss and come & go as I please.

Much love to you and Papa and the rest, from Grace

Grace mentioned that she rode horses and played volleyball. The Commission on Training Camp Activities devised a wide-ranging athletic program for soldiers. The CTCA promoted competi-

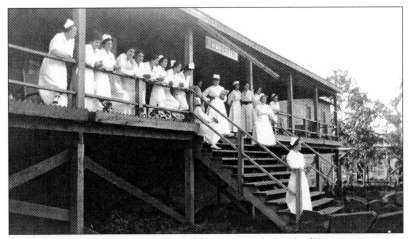

Grace snapped this photo of the Camp Pike nurses on the porch of their quarters. (19)

tive sports for physical fitness and to strengthen the instinctive fighting spirit. Coaches offered organized athletics such as boxing, football, baseball, wrestling, soccer, swimming, tennis, cross-country running, volleyball, and gymnastics. Athletic directors scheduled intramural games, especially for baseball, between teams of various cantonments.[13]

Meeting "Secretary of War Baker's wife," who toured the operating rooms, delighted Grace. The woman she described as "unassuming" was Elizabeth Leopold Baker, the wife of Newton Diehl Baker, secretary of war.

By June 30, 1918, shortly before Grace received her orders, over four thousand nurses served in Europe. More than one thousand awaited embarkation or were en route to the mobilization station.[14]

Camp Pike - July 10, '18

Dear Mamma & Papa,

This is my last letter to you from Camp Pike. I leave tomorrow for New York, and then very soon – overseas. I am very glad to go and whatever happens, everything is all right. I haven't the least fear or worry in the world. Am ready for anything. Will write you from New York if I can, and as often as I am allowed to, overseas.

It is now past midnight so I must go to bed. You understand of course that you must not tell for some time, that I am
on my way, as it is dangerous for us to have it known. I shall
give you all the information I can.

My best friend, Miss Edith Muir, and I received our orders from Washington together. Tell Nell [her sister-in-law]
that I got her letter & enjoyed it. And now good-night. My
best love to you all, Grace

Grace entrained at Camp Pike on July 12, 1918, to "proceed
without delay" to the nurses' mobilization station at the Holley
Hotel, Washington Square West, New York City. The army directed
her to report, upon arrival, to the commanding general, port of
embarkation, Hoboken, New Jersey, for further orders.[15]

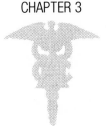

CHAPTER 3

Going "Over There"

We drill every day just like the soldiers ...
am a real soldier now.[1]
—Grace Anderson

World War I dominated the activities in New York City when Grace Anderson reported for mobilization in July 1918. Twelve years earlier well-wishers bid bon voyage to Grace as she boarded a steamer for a vacation in Europe. During wartime, troopships slipped out of the harbor without fanfare in the darkness of night.

In July, the busiest month for departures, more than 300,000 American soldiers crossed the Atlantic. Most of the over 1.6 million troops, who sailed overseas from April through October 1918, embarked at the New York harbor piers.[2]

Thousands of soldiers drilled in the city and at nearby camps as they waited for their orders. Draft-age men carried their registration cards everywhere in case of surprise "slacker raids" at workplaces, train stations, ballparks, homes, restaurants, union halls, hotels, and theaters.[3]

Posters, pamphlets, and advertising from the Committee on Public Information blanketed the area. Four Minute Men inspired

attendees at public events with talks about country and cause. Red
Cross volunteers knitted sweaters and socks and made thousands of
surgical dressings for the armed forces.

Movie theaters screened war-related newsreels and documenta-
ries. D.W. Griffith's successful film, *Hearts of the World*, opened in
New York in April and ran for six months. A gripping plot favoring
the Allies and some footage shot on the battlefields brought the
Great War to the home front.[3]

Some of the Manhattan hotels, where Grace and other voyagers
stayed in 1906, became mobilization locations. On July 14 she lined
up for her Certificate of Identity, tags, and uniforms at the Holley

Grace and other nurses received their Certificates of Identity at the
Nurses Mobilization Station in New York City. (20)

Hotel Station, Washington Square West, and the Nurses Mobilization Station on Madison Avenue.

> New York, NY - July 16, '18
> Dear Mamma & Papa,
>
> Have arrived safely and my address will be in care of Base Hospital Unit 115, 120 Madison Ave., New York City. I am seeing New York, all right, too. Have already been from the mansions on upper 5th Ave., to the Italian quarter & Chinatown.
>
> We drill every day just like soldiers – a regular army officer is drilling us, and he says we learn about ten times as quick as the men. Yesterday afternoon he said we accomplished three times as much as he expected.
>
> We will soon have our uniforms. Will try to send you a picture. Am a real soldier now. If anything happens to me, you Mamma, are to use your share of my insurance for yourself as long as you live. Then anyone you want can share the benefit. Papa can do as he wants about his share too.
>
> Love, Grace

The army considered Grace, who liked being "a real soldier now," a full member of the armed forces. However, the Red Cross furnished the nurses' uniforms and equipment. Following the war, the government reimbursed the Red Cross.[4]

Military and nursing leaders disagreed about the status of the Army Nurse Corps. The army granted the ANC only paramilitary status and expected the women to exercise authority without rank. The ANC believed their demanding responsibilities merited the rank of officer with equal pay and benefits. When the army rejected the plea for equal rank, the ANC requested relative rank. The nurses would be called lieutenant or captain and have respect and authority but without the same benefits.[5]

The ANC persevered in arguing their case for equal or relative rank. Meanwhile, the dedicated nurses in Europe gave patients the best care medical science could offer. Grace, undeterred by the on-going controversy, drilled "every day just like soldiers."

As a member of Base No. 115, Grace belonged to a military unit of the American Expeditionary Forces, the army and marines in France. Nurses at 127 AEF base hospitals aided the majority of over 1.3 million patients admitted to base and camp hospitals and convalescent camps. Although troops hospitalized with illness, wounds, and non-battle injuries included Allies, patients were mostly doughboys, the nickname for U.S. infantrymen in World War I. In the base hospital system, which functioned from May 1917 through June 1919, the maximum beds available in November 1918 ranged from 192,964 for normal and crisis expansion to 230,756 for emergency.[6]

In the early years of the Great War, while Grace studied nursing at Northwestern Hospital in Minneapolis, the base hospitals had their genesis. Myron T. Herrick, U.S. ambassador to France, asked Dr. George W. Crile, a prominent surgeon, to serve in the American Ambulance Hospital in Paris. Crile, a professor of surgery at Western Reserve University in Cleveland, advocated medical preparedness in the eventuality of future entry in World War I.[7]

Crile led his surgical personnel from Lakeside Hospital in Cleveland to Paris in January 1915. For three months they treated casualties at Neuilly and gained valuable military surgery experience. In October Crile presented the concept of base hospital units in Boston at the Symposium on Military Surgery, Clinical Congress of Surgeons of North America. Crile proposed forming the units at recognized institutions. In his opinion, medical staffs with similar professional training, who worked together regularly, would provide the most efficient medical service in the war.[7]

William C. Gorgas, U.S. Army surgeon general, enthusiastically approved the preparedness plan but the peacetime army lacked the necessary funds for the project. Gorgas sought the assistance of the Red Cross, a civilian organization, to implement the base hospital system. The Red Cross agreed to collaborate with the army in establishing fifty hospitals and raise money with supervision from the surgeon general's office. American volunteers, who helped the British and French overseas from 1914 to 1917, shared their insights and medical expertise.[7]

During those three years of the war before U.S. involvement, the Army Medical Department undertook medical preparedness, which the nation's medical profession supported. Thousands of physicians and surgeons, bacteriologists, epidemiologists, and public health experts would serve in the army voluntarily if they were needed. Consequently, the army was better prepared to give excellent medical service in World War I than at the start of any previous wars.[7]

The army designated base hospitals, located a safe distance from combat zones, for more extensive and definitive treatment. These fixed facilities, the foundation of AEF medical services, would operate in conjunction with battlefield first aid, dressing stations, ambulances, and hospital trains as well as field, mobile, evacuation, camp, and convalescent hospitals.[7]

Medical groups, professional organizations, colleges, and universities across the country participated in fund-raising. All parties understood that if the United States engaged in the hostilities, the military would take over the base hospitals.[7]

Early in 1916 civilian hospitals and university medical schools began putting together medical personnel and equipment for base units. New York Hospital and Harvard University produced the first ones in February 1916. The same year Base No. 4, Dr. Crile's Cleveland team, and thirteen others developed.[8]

By the time Grace graduated as a registered nurse in late 1916 and joined the Northwestern Hospital staff in Minneapolis, news of the base hospitals had spread throughout the nation. In 1917 the majority of the first fifty units organized. In May, the month after Congress declared war, the University of Minnesota formed Base No. 26 in Minneapolis. All the war-related medical activity in the city where she lived intrigued Grace. However, she wanted to complete her anesthetist course before deciding how to "do her bit."[8]

Additional university units included Emory, Atlanta; Northwestern, Chicago; Tulane, New Orleans, and the Universities of

California, Maryland, Nebraska, Oregon, Pennsylvania, Virginia, and Washington. Other prominent hospitals were Bellevue, Mount Sinai, and Presbyterian, New York; Johns Hopkins, Baltimore; St. Luke and Michael Reese, Chicago, and Good Samaritan, Los Angeles.[8]

Medical students signed up with the Johns Hopkins Hospital Base No. 18 and other units. Thirty-two of the Base No. 18 enlisted men, all third-year medical school students, planned to finish their last scholastic year in France, receive their degrees, and be commissioned in the Medical Reserve Corps.[8]

In May and early June of 1917, before the doughboys arrived, the AEF assigned six base units to the British Expeditionary Forces at BEF general hospitals. They were the first American army units to fly the U.S. flag in France. Dr. Crile's unit at the BEF hospital in Rouen was the first AEF detachment to reach Europe. Eleven others followed in 1917 and the rest in 1918.[8]

Grace's Base No. 115 and all the units had one hundred nurses, thirty-five Medical Corps officers, two hundred enlisted men and some civilian employees such as dieticians and technicians. The men of Base No. 115 organized in June 1918 at Camp May, New Jersey, as part of the second group of eighty base hospitals. During 1918 the units, consisting of officers and enlisted men, came mainly from nationwide military camps, with over half from Camp Greenleaf, Fort Oglethorpe, Georgia.[8]

Base No. 115 and the second group usually progressed through organization, mobilization, and training to arrival in Europe in three months. For units assembled prior to U.S entry in the conflict, the time period was four months to more than a year. Base units trained for two to four months. Nearly half of the originally planned units, which were numbered up to 238, never became base hospitals in France. Most of them never mobilized before the armistice and some were reassigned to other hospitals.[8]

Grace and her sister nurses of Base No. 115 "came from every corner of our land." Yet they possessed the same mind and spirit, as expressed in the lyrics of their song, sent in Grace's July 22 letter.

New York City - July 22, '18

Dear Mamma & Papa,

You want to know all I can tell you about going overseas. Well, the unit #115 that I am with is supposed to be a brain surgery unit. They call it the "head" unit. We expect to be stationed about seven miles from Verdun, but of course we know nothing definite about that.

We are very nearly equipped now. We haven't got our uniforms but we have had all our fittings and expect them in a few days. We got our passports or our identification papers today. We wear silver tags around our necks on silver chains, and on mine it says - Grace M. Anderson Army Nurse Corps U.S.A. Base Hospital Unit #115. If anything happens to us this one tag will be sent to you. The other left on me.

Our suits are dark blue Norfolk style, serge, and very nice. Our big coats (top coats), we can wear right over our suits and they match the suits in style & color. We have one blue flannel waist, two blue silk waists and two white wash waists. Our shoes are like the soldiers only nicer. We have two pairs of tan & one of black. Our gloves match our shoes. Our hats are blue sailors, straw for summer, velour for winter. Our indoor uniforms are gray with white collars, cuffs, & aprons & caps. Our out of door uniforms are very good looking & splendid quality.

It is costing us a good deal to get all the little things we need. Am spending more than I expected but after all now is the time for me to get the good of my money. Will save & make up after the war if I'm alive. If I'm not, it won't matter anyway.

We drill every day just like the soldiers and I tell you it is hard work. There isn't much to tell you that I haven't told. Ask me if there is anything you want to know.

When we get ready to sail everything will be very quiet. We will leave our quarters without any luggage, and when we are on board, our boat will slip away some night. If anything happens, I've a little money in the Northwestern National Bank in Minneapolis. What is left is for you, Mamma.

Will send my clothes home in a cheap suitcase. I haven't very much left. Thought maybe you would enjoy our Unit song. Here it is, the words anyway. The nurses are very patriotic & enthusiastic.

> Every Sammy who is going over there!
> Every Jackie on the sea,
> Has pledged his life to fight for liberty
> And so have we.
> We'll take our chance with them in France.
> When General Pershing calls us to do our bit
> We'll welcome the opportunity.
> If there's any comfort we can show,
> Just tell about it, we'll be glad to know.
> We're "Head" Unit, No. One Fifteen, Boys
> One fifteen is coming just one hundred strong
> From every corner of our land.
> Hold the Fort! We'll soon be with you, Boys,
> To share your joys, your sorrow, pain and everything.
> We're glad you're there, we're glad that we are coming, too
> To help you to win the victory.
> Pride of America, we're with you,
> All of our strength we'll gladly give you.
> Wait for us, Unit One fifteen, Boys.

Will write once more before I sail. Hope everyone is well. Give them all my love. Grace

Grace pointed out they would "slip away some night." The soldiers departed secretly due to German submarine attacks in the Atlantic. The German high command thought U-boats could force an early surrender of the Allies by cutting off their supplies on cargo ships and by stopping the American armed forces from crossing to Europe. The unrestricted submarine campaign sunk nearly nine hundred thousand

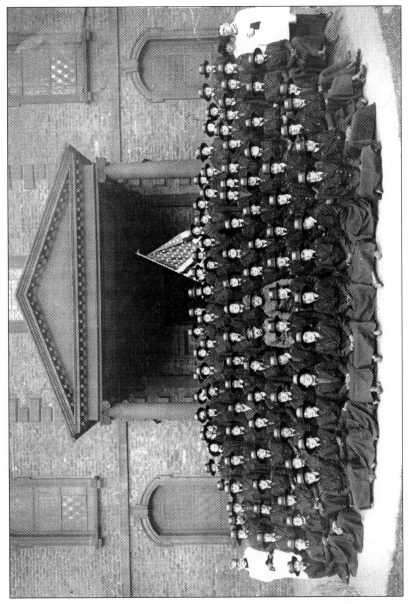

The one hundred nurses of Base Hospital No. 115 gathered at St. Paul's Church in New York City. "Me" with an arrow pointed to Grace, sixth from the right in the fourth row from the bottom. (21)

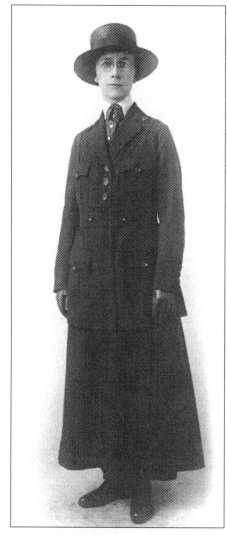

Grace described her U.S. Army Nurse Corps uniform in detail in her July 22, 1918 letter home. This photo is also on the back cover. (22)

tons of Allied cargo per month and destroyed hundreds of vessels.[9]

After the United States entered the conflict, the American Navy helped the British decrease the effectiveness of U-boats with the convoy system. To dramatically reduce shipping losses, several merchant ships grouped together. Destroyers and other anti-submarine vessels escorted them through the war zone. The U. S. Navy escorted most of the trans-Atlantic troopship convoys and operated cargo vessels that transported more than seven million tons of supplies and thousands of horses and mules to France.[9,10]

Although the Royal Navy primarily battled the U-boats, the U.S. Navy reinforced the British fleet. The Americans significantly supported the Allies with destroyers, battleships, submarines, and other vessels in the naval effort of anti-submarine patrols, convoy escorts, and mine barrage laying. A U.S. naval aviation force assisted the escorting and submarine hunting.[9,10]

Three quarters of the doughboys embarked in New York and the rest left from additional United States and Canadian ports. They voyaged to British and French ports with most of them landing in Liverpool or Brest.[11]

Grace's Base No. 115 and many hospital units traveled from New York/Hoboken to France by way of England. In Liverpool they entrained for the trip to Southampton. At night they boarded British cross-channel steamers and U.S. naval transports and landed at Le Havre the next morning. Others sailed from New York/Hoboken or Newport News to Brest or St. Nazaire. Some units split up, journeyed on different convoy vessels, and reassembled in England or France.[11]

Although the United States lacked adequate shipping capacity for the over two million troops, the country carried more than nine hundred thousand on U.S. Navy and non-military transports. Those ships included German and Austrian steamers, seized when the war began. The British transported over one million. French, Italian, and other foreign vessels handled the remainder.[11]

The hospital units joined the armed forces on over sixty-five different ships. Some of them voyaged on Germany's high-speed *Leviathan*, seized by the United States. More than one hundred thousand troops traveled on the *Leviathan*, known as the world's largest liner in 1914.[11]

The men of Base No.115 stayed in the United States to conclude mobilization and equipping. As Grace and the nurses in her unit prepared to leave on July 30, they heard about accidents that happened in or near New York harbor in 1917.[12]

On May 20, the day after Northwestern University Base No. 12 departed, a gun of the *Mongolia* misfired during target practice. Shell fragments accidentally and tragically killed two nurses and wounded a third. The *Mongolia* returned and set out again for Europe on May 24.[12]

In July New York Post-Graduate Hospital Base No. 8 embarked on the *Saratoga* and the *Panama* rammed the ship. Although everyone disembarked safely from the badly damaged vessel, they lost medical equipment and personal belongings. After a delay for re-equipping, they sailed on the *Finland*.[12]

The nurses knew that going overseas, barring any unforeseen circumstances, usually took almost two weeks. The Atlantic passage could be grueling with rough weather, seasickness, and the constant threat of submarine attacks.

Grace's steamer trip with her parents in 1906, described by her mother in a letter to a friend, contrasted sharply with her 1918 wartime experience.

> We had a beautiful voyage. The weather was lovely. It was quite cold a couple days but that was on account of our passing a number of icebergs. There were 1,300 passengers, six hundred men of the crew. One hundred of these were waiters in the dining salon ...We saw a number of whale spouting water but they were some distance from the steamer.[13]

Crowded troopships, with blackouts to avoid enemy sightings, replaced earlier luxurious voyages. Activities ranged from frequent lifeboat safety drills and military formations to singing, religious services, and sometimes band concerts. By keeping their minds and bodies active, Grace and her sister nurses relieved their stress about U-boats and dangers awaiting them in Europe.[14]

Grace's mother received a formal note with "A Message to You from His Majesty King George" printed on the envelope. The message, under the Windsor Castle royal emblem, said:

> Soldiers of the United States, the people of the British Isles welcome you on your way to take your stand beside the Armies of many Nations now fighting in the Old World the great battle for human freedom.
>
> The Allies will gain new heart & spirit in your company. I wish that I could shake the hand of each one of you & bid you God speed on your mission.
>
> (signed) George R.I. April 1918[15]

King George V of the United Kingdom tried to maintain national unity and morale. The king frequently visited the fighting

WINDSOR CASTLE.

Soldiers of the United States, the people of the British Isles welcome you on your way to take your stand beside the Armies of many Nations now fighting in the Old World the great battle for human freedom.
The Allies will gain new heart & spirit in your company.
I wish that I could shake the hand of each one of you & bid you God-speed on your mission.

George R.I.

April 1918.

Ellen Anderson, Grace's mother, received this note sent to the American troops by King George V of the United Kingdom. (23)

men and the injured in hospitals. Grace disembarked in England on about the same day, August 12, as the postmark on the king's note.

Before the doughboys departed they filled out and addressed postcards, held by the Red Cross until a cable from Europe confirmed a safe crossing. Grace's postcard to her parents stated: "The ship on which I sailed has arrived safely overseas. Name - Grace M. Anderson; Organization - U.S.A. Base Hospital Unit #115, American Expeditionary Forces." Grace wrote her first letter from "over there" to her brother, Clarence, at the Mayo Clinic.

U.S. Base Hospital Unit #115
American Expeditionary Forces
Somewhere – Sometime in 1918!
Clarence Dear –

Just a line from "this other side." We landed in ——— and hope to stay here a while but do not know what the orders will be.

I'd love to write you about our trip over, but by the time all the "don'ts" are eliminated there is very little to tell. But wait till I come home. I'll tell all the things I can't tell now. It is very interesting and wonderful to see how things are managed.

Have only a minute to write now. Write often as you can to me. My address will be, U.S. Base Hospital Unit 115 American

Expeditionary Forces. Be sure to spell the words out. And don't be surprised if some of your letters don't reach me. Keep writing just the same. You will get my letters easier than I'll get yours.

We've heard some wonderful tales from people who have been "there." I think I'll be able to write more about things when we are on land. We had some rather rough weather but I seemed to get my sea legs at once and was not sick. As you see, our mail goes without postage as "soldier's mail." You know of course that your letters to me only require a three-cent stamp. Oceans of love, Grace

August 1918
Dear "Folks,"

A letter to you all from overseas! We had a pleasant trip, and enjoyed it in spite of the dangers. I'm not allowed to tell you much about it, but will say it was a long trip and we are required to wear life preservers all the time.

Also, we nurses are provided with rubber suits, which keep one afloat and warm & dry for forty-eight hours. We haven't needed them but I want you to know what the Red Cross does for us, even to furnishing these rubber suits. No one on board has them but the nurses. These suits are complete even to rubber caps & whistles around our necks so we can call for help. The feet are weighted so a person stays in an upright position in the water even if unconscious. The Red Cross furnished our outfit, we never could have afforded to buy it ourselves. I'm sure it would have cost us three hundred dollars.

You will get two suitcases by express, one mine and one my chum's. I explained, I think, that at the last minute she couldn't get it thru to Canada. If you have any trouble, just hold Miss Muir's suitcase there. Mamma, she has some furs and a wool suit. You'll see that the moths don't get in, won't you.

I was called so suddenly when I was called, even while expecting it, I wasn't expecting it. That sounds funny but it's true. I had them send you a picture of our Unit taken in New York at the old St. Paul's church – the church George Washington used to attend. We had our dedication service for our unit flag in this church.

For, if you please, we have a very beautiful flag, which we carry when our unit marches, same as the soldiers have. You see the flag in the picture, at the back. I hope you received the picture. Also, we had some pictures taken in uniform the evening before we left New York. We left so soon we didn't even see them, but a friend said he would get them and send them to you. You must try to write to me often, because you can be sure not every letter will reach me. Give my love to all the family. Am sorry I can't tell you all the interesting things I want to tell about, but they will have to keep till I get home. We are not even supposed to give dates. Best love, Grace

Grace wanted to tell her family several "interesting things," such as her unexpected adventure. She crossed the English Channel on a submarine, one of seven U.S. Navy boats that assisted Allied submarines in keeping sea lanes open. Starting in early 1918, American submarines became active in the Irish Sea, English Channel, and other coastal waters. Apparently great numbers of arriving troops overloaded the usual transports. Much to Grace's delight, a submarine carried some nurses because the AEF desperately needed them.[16]

Grace arrived overseas six days after the AEF cabled a request for absolute priority on transports for medical organizations, including 2,312 nurses. The increased involvement of the United States in combat nearly exhausted the Medical Department's personnel resources. Grace was among one thousand nurses who reached France in August 1918.[17]

At the Vichy Hospital Center she learned that the men of Base No. 115 were still on the Atlantic. As a result, the AEF issued temporary orders to Grace and most of her unit's nurses. Changes in duty stations were fairly common. Some medical personnel temporarily worked at Pontanezen, a camp near the port of Brest, where many doughboys rested before continuing to their destinations. Other base unit doctors and nurses moved to field and mobile hospitals near the front lines during major battles.[18]

After a seventeen-day journey on sea and land, Grace welcomed having two days in Vichy to catch up on laundry, letters, and sleep. Grace, her best friend, Edith, and other Base No. 115 nurses received the same orders for duty at Base Hospital No. 17 in Dijon.[19]

On August 18 the women boarded the first of two trains that would take them to their new assignment, closer to the war zone. Their promise to "our boys" to "share your joys, sorrow, pain and everything"[20] allayed any apprehension they felt. Grace and her sister nurses were ready and willing to "take our chance with them in France"[21] and go wherever necessary to care for the sick and injured soldiers.

CHAPTER 4

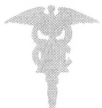

Healing
"Our Boys"

*Our boys are the finest & best in the world. I love them all
and am happy working for them. You never saw such
patience and grit as they have.*[1]
—Grace Anderson

As the train from Vichy approached Paris, Grace watched an air raid darken the City of Light. The ominous welcome introduced her to the hostilities of bomber squadrons far above trenches of the western front. When Grace registered at the Hotel Continental as a U.S. Army nurse, her overnight stay in wartime Paris contrasted with her visit as a tourist more than a decade earlier.

In the Aisne-Marne sector, only seventy-five miles northeast of the Eiffel Tower, Allies and Germans fought in the Second Battle of the Marne. After the Germans attacked on July 15, divisions of the American Expeditionary Forces, under French command, joined with the Allies in a counter offensive that raged for a month.[2]

Grace journeyed south via rail to Dijon and arrived August 19, a day after the Allies launched the Oise-Aisne offensive. Within four weeks they achieved their first victorious offensive of 1918. Over 250,000 AEF men, who participated in both defense and

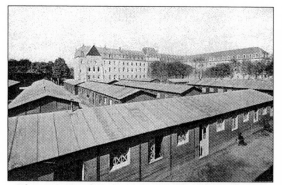

The army issued Grace new orders for temporary duty at Base Hospital No. 17 in Dijon, France. (24)

advances during the Second Battle of the Marne, helped turn the tide of World War I in favor of the Allies.[2]

Prior to the war, Dijon's medieval art treasures and architecture attracted travelers. The centuries-old town, in the zone of advance, was about eighty miles from the front lines. U.S. Army medical personnel and the injured, transported by trains and ambulances, replaced previous visitors.

Harper Hospital in Detroit organized Base No. 17, Grace's temporary duty station. The army's difficulties in finding adequate facilities led to challenging beginnings for Base No. 17, one of the early units functioning in the summer of 1917. Assigned the French army's Hospital St. Ignace, the unit waited two weeks while the French evacuated their patients. The Americans, unable to postpone any longer, started accepting their troops before the French released the facility to the U.S. commanding officer. The hospital outgrew its original space and expanded by acquiring a large stone French seminary a few miles away at Plombiers.[3]

The army located base units in French hospitals and seminaries as well as an array of old stone, masonry, and cement structures mixed with new ones. The teams offered medical care in French military barracks, schools, old monasteries, hotels of all sizes, villas, estates, private residences, gymnasiums, and factories.[3]

At Bazoilles, Johns Hopkins Hospital Base No. 18, attended soldiers at an estate property with a stone hunting lodge, groups of out buildings, numerous new frame structures, and twenty-five acres of forested land. In Chateauroux, New York Hospital Base No. 9 occupied several new wooden wards and an insane asylum, formerly used as a French military hospital. The convalescent patients tended an eighteen-acre farm, where they raised fresh vegetables for the mess halls.[3]

Before the base units reached France, the AEF scouted locations using lists of available buildings provided by the French. The military selected sites accessible by trains from the front and the rear, with terrain suitable for new construction, satisfactory available structures, and a good water supply. The AEF leased schools, hotels, and other buildings, not previously hospitals, from the French army.[3]

The hospital units counted on the Army Corps of Engineers to handle their building projects. The movement and supply of the AEF in France relied on the massive construction achievements of the corps. The engineers harvested timber, operated sawmills, and produced board lumber, railroad ties, and timber piles. They built port facilities, roads, railroad tracks, bridges, barracks, gas tanks, storage depots, laundries, and airdromes.[4]

Eight hundred thousand pounds of bread, baked each day at one of the engineers' electrically run bakeries, helped feed the troops. Their over two-thousand-foot Loire River bridge was the longest one made by Americans in France.[4]

The corps prepared existing structures for medical use by cleaning and remodeling or converting entire interiors. They built wooden barracks and hospitals, mostly of one thousand beds and also five or six thousand beds.[4]

Some places transformed easier than others. In Toul, Base No. 45 from the Medical College of Virginia took over Caserne La Marche. The group of four-story buildings, without plumbing or electricity, called for extensive overhauling. The corps needed to construct fifty-two wooden structures in a park near the center of Limoges for Base No. 13 from Presbyterian Hospital in Chicago. In contrast, at Le Mont Dore, Base No. 93 from Camp Lewis, Wash., moved into the Sarciron, the largest and most modern hotel in the city. In two days the unit admitted cases.[4]

Often medical personnel resided in fascinating quarters like the former palace in Dijon, where Grace and other nurses lived.

Base Hospital No. 17 - Aug. 24, '18

Dear Mamma & Papa,

We are stationed temporarily in a hospital of about fifteen hundred beds. We like the work very much. When the fresh cases are brought in, it means work steady for a good many hours at a time, so everyone rests when they can.

I'm not allowed to tell you very much but we are about in the middle of France, at Dijon. Our trip over was uneventful except for air raids. There was one going on in Paris as we entered the city. We watched it from the distance as we came along on the train.

When we pulled into the station every place was pitch dark and we had to stumble along as best we could. We were finally taken to the Hotel Continental. Very little damage was done and no one seems to pay much attention to the air raids, as far as being frightened goes.

From what we hear, the Germans must be pretty much up against it. They are, when they go up against our troops. Our boys are so quick, the English and the French tell us that is what counts. They are all enthusiastic about our boys.

My love to everyone, most for yourselves, Grace

In June, two months before Grace witnessed an air raid in Paris, the U.S. Air Service demonstrated its combat capability at Chateau-Thierry. In September American aerial operations at St. Mihiel turned that battle into a significant event in U.S. military aviation history. Col. William ("Billy") Mitchell, who planned the air phase, assembled and led more than 1,400 American, British, French, and Italian aircraft in the largest single air force in World War I.[5]

Following St. Mihiel, American airmen kept increasing their aerial warfare. Aggressive pursuit pilots gained fame for their dogfights. Observation and bomber crews flew critical and valuable reconnaissance and bombardment missions. In spite of their bomber squadrons' big losses in men and aircraft, Americans continued flying missions until the Armistice. The U.S. Air Service, which ended the war with 45 squadrons and 740 airplanes, contributed mean-ingfully to the Allied effort.[5]

Base Hospital No. 17 - Sept. 1, '18
Dear Mamma & Papa,

It is just a month since I left New York and here I am nicely settled in an American hospital in France. Things are much better than I expected to find them. Our food is good and there is plenty of it.

We have quarters which are not exactly luxurious, having nothing but a cot each and a few chairs, but we are warm enough and well fed, so you see you do not need to worry about me.

Our soldier boys are fine and we love to do all we can for them. They are always laughing and joking away their troubles. There is very little trouble with them and no complaining.

The sickest man we have in the ward is a Pole about forty-five years old. He has two sons in the army too. He is just recovering from pneumonia as well as a very painful wound in his leg. One of the nurses said to him, "Well, John, I guess you wish you had never come into the army." And he answered "No, I fight for a good country, a free country, I got to go to the front again when I get well!" How is that for spirit?

Our boys are making a great impression here, and they are such fine fellows we are all proud of them. They are making things hum, aren't they?

It is very quiet here. There are a great many places of his-torical interest to visit and, as French towns go, is supposed to be a good one. Much love to all, Grace

Base Hospital No. 17 - Sept. 8, '18
Dear Mamma,

Will you please order me some of those woven name tapes? My sewing case and everything in it was stolen the other day and all my name tapes were in it. I was in a store and had laid my things down in front of me while I looked at something and a little French girl about 8 years old grabbed my bundle & ran. Poor youngsters. I hope it does her some good. There was about five dollars worth of stuff in the package.

I haven't had any mail yet and I appreciate how the soldiers feel when they don't get letters. It takes so long to get mail that unless people write right along the intervals between letters are very long.

I have to dress much warmer here already. I guess it will be a cold winter all right. You get as much war news in the papers as I can give you, but I can say everything is just as bright as the papers say. Have seen lots of German prisoners both in France & in England. Write often as you can. Love, Grace

Base Hospital No. 17 - Sept. 9, '18
Dear Clarence,

I hope you are writing to me often because I'm pretty lonesome, and you can't imagine how we all watch for the mail. I haven't had a single letter yet.

We live in an old house, supposedly a palace, and from the mosaic floors and the marble, etc., it at least must have been the home of wealthy people. Down under ground there are cellars, dungeons and underground passages running halfway across the town and connecting with the real palace.

The old churches are very beautiful and one of them has a tower with chimes that are run by automatics – figures of a man, a woman and two children. It always makes me smile to see it. Wish you could see all these interesting things.

This morning I had to go to a French post office to get a money order. It took fully an hour to manage it between my French and their English. One is quite helpless without a command of the French language. Am studying again and hope to learn it – in self defense!

We are not very busy right now, the hospital is not nearly full. There isn't much to write about, that I feel I would be allowed to write. Conditions are not as bad as I expected, tho of course we are roughing it as far as living goes. The food we nurses have is the same as the boys have, so I know what I'm talking about when I say the boys' food is good. And most of them say it is still better up at the front, except at times of big battles, of course.

Be sure and write often, brother dear. It is sometimes two months before your letters reach their destination.

Much love, Grace

Soon after Grace wrote Clarence about Base No. 17 not being full, the workload soared. A flood of wounded from the Second Battle of the Marne, which had thirty thousand casualties,[6] followed by patients from the Meuse-Argonne offensive, inundated the hospital. More than one million Americans participated in the Meuse-

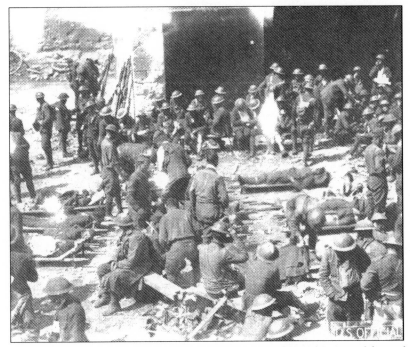

In the AEF medical handling procedure in France, wounded troops received first aid at stations like this one of the First Division, immediately back of the front line trenches at Missy-aux-Bois.(25)

Argonne battle from September 26 to November 11, 1918. During the biggest AEF operation and victory, 26,277 AEF men were killed and 95,786 were wounded.[7]

The overwhelming numbers of injured far surpassed the previous civilian nursing experiences of Grace, her best friend Edith, and other nurses. They feared they might fail to meet the war's demands. But the bravery of the doughboys inspired them to prove they could handle multiple tasks with increasing efficiency. Although Grace worked fourteen to eighteen hours a day, she downplayed her stressful shifts and the suffering around her in letters home. Instead she praised "our boys" for their courage, spirit, and positive attitude.

Base No. 17, closer to the front lines, functioned as an evacuation hospital during major battles when casualties were too numerous for field hospitals to manage. In response to the predicted number of battle casualties, nurses implemented crisis expansion by doubling the bed capacity.[8]

Masses of ill and injured tested the nurses' adaptability. They squeezed extra beds and cots into hallways, crowded wards, and

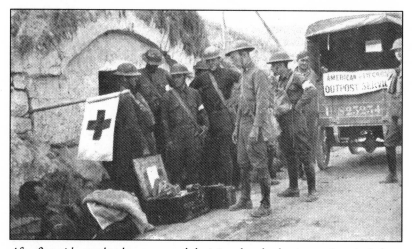

After first aid, stretcher-bearers moved the injured to the dressing station. Ambulance Company No. 111, Twenty-eighth Division, operated this dressing station near St. Gilles. (26)

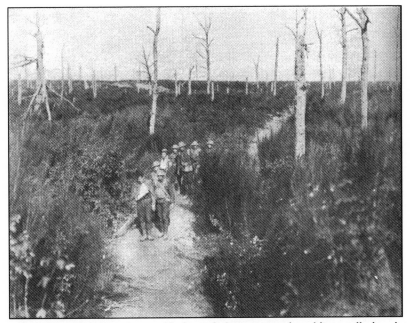

When the roads became impassable for ambulances or trucks, soldiers walked to the dressing station, as these men did in the Argonne Forest.(27)

attics. They lined up mattresses on the floors. If possible, the Corps of Engineers erected Nissen huts and marquee tents for the overflow of patients.[8]

In crisis times Base No. 17 received troops directly from the front. In a December letter Grace told Clarence, her brother, what they faced. "We worked harder there than they did at the front because we worked steady all the time and at the front they had a let up when there wasn't a drive on. And the boys we got, had only had first aid, you know, when they came to us.

"Our convoys always came in at night, so the day forces had to stay up and help take care of the arrivals. The last convoy I got before I left that hospital were all stretcher cases and such a sight I never want to see again."

The stretcher cases shivered from trauma and blood loss and shook with shell shock. Soldiers suffered injuries primarily from artillery. Flying metal fragments of shells killed troops suddenly or hurt them dreadfully by embedding in them from ankles to skulls. Sharp, jagged pieces shattered or severed bones, muscles, vessels or nerves and paralyzed some men.[9]

Artillery as well as machine guns, rifles, and the poison gases of chemical warfare left soldiers writhing in agony with legs, arms, and jaws blown away. Doughboys had destroyed limbs, split heads, and skin burned and blistered by mustard gas. Some got entangled in barbed wire defenses that ripped and tore their flesh. Phosgene inhalation caused fluid in the lungs, coughing, choking, and ultimately suffocation.[9]

Bombardments stopped litter-bearers from reaching blood-soaked soldiers who took cover in trenches filled with mud, lice, rats, mosquitoes, flies, and disease. The delay caused severe infections, loss of limbs, and illnesses including pneumonia, influenza, and dysentery.[9]

Doctors and nurses persevered to the point of exhaustion dealing with the ghastly horrors the conflagration inflicted on once whole and healthy young men. Because they treated thousands of injuries, medical teams rapidly developed and improved their methods to save lives.

The Americans who had non-mortal wounds numbered 204,002. Deaths from injuries, disease, and other causes were 116,516. Of the 53,402 battle deaths, the majority were killed in action and about 13,000 died of wounds.[10]

Since antibiotics did not exist, doctors and nurses fought infection in gaping wounds with tetanus antitoxin, debridement, and irrigation. Surgeons opened wounds, removed tiny pieces of dirt, metal, bone, and clothing, and then excised the contaminated or dead tissue. Nurses irrigated the open injury with antiseptic, usually Dakin's solution, using perforated rubber tubes. Additional antiseptic treatments and re-dressings followed the first sterile dressing. A surgeon sutured the wound when a bacteriological examination determined that it was free of germs.[11]

Grace and her sister nurses called on their resourcefulness to help soldiers who had injuries requiring irrigation and also shattered limbs or compound fractures. They prepared a variety of devices for patient comfort and care by themselves or assisted by corpsmen and orderlies. Nurses combined bed frames (Bradford or Balkan) with extensions for traction of broken legs, hung bottles of Dakin's solution for irrigation, placed hammocks under shoulders or backs, and adjusted ropes and pulleys. They also made on-the-spot inventions.[11]

The casualties that Grace and Base No. 17 aided usually progressed through a life-saving handling procedure that began near the front lines. Army nurses worked in casualty clearing stations and field, mobile, and evacuation hospitals in the advance section. Normally only severe cases were transferred to base hospitals, the last step. Then recovered doughboys returned to duty. Some went to convalescent camps and others, who were permanently disabled or seriously diseased, became unfit for military duty. When they could be transported, they boarded ships for the United States and general hospitals like Walter Reed in Washington, D.C.[12]

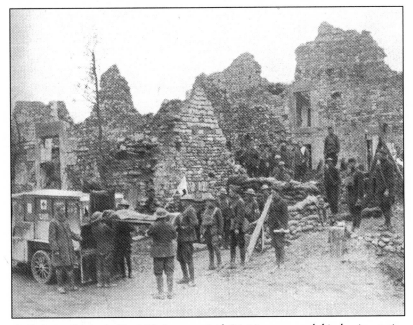

Ambulance Company No. 316, Seventy-ninth Division, operated this dressing station in Les Eparges, Meuse. This photo is also on the front cover. (28)

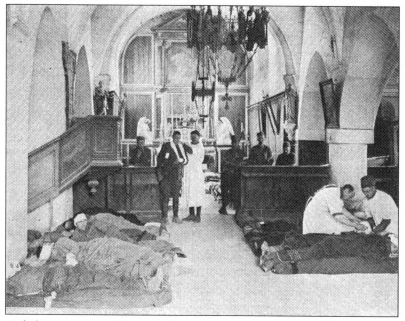

Ambulances transported the injured from the dressing stations to the field hospitals. Field Hospital No. 1, Second Division, used the church at Bezu-Le-Guery as a ward. (29)

Initially troops received first aid on the battlefield. Then they walked or litter-bearers carried them, sometimes in pounding rain, to a battalion or regimental first aid station for further emergency attention. Removing a stretcher and one soldier from a muddy battlefield sometimes required six men. Diagnosis tags, tied on to patients, had their name, an abbreviation such as G.S.W. for gunshot wound, location (arm, leg, abdomen), and a medical officer's name.[12]

Stretcher-bearers moved the doughboys, or they walked, to the dressing station, less than two miles from the lines, where doctors attended them. Depending on road conditions, the men rode in horse-drawn or motor ambulances to the field hospital, two to four miles from the front. Litter-bearers pushed or pulled contrivances with wheels to transport the wounded on roads where the Germans shelled trucks and ambulances.[12]

Triage sorted casualties according to urgency and chance for survival. Surgeons performed emergency operations for abdominal, chest, and other serious wounds. Doctors sent cases to special hospitals designated for gassed victims. Medical staffs offered specific treatment for eye conditions, skin burns, and lung irritation due to exposure to toxic warfare gasses. Ambulances conveyed other soldiers to the mobile hospital.[12]

The staff recorded the patient's name, regiment, rank, nature and date of the wound or injury, and gave anti-tetanus injections. After surgery evaluation, some troops went to an operating room and the rest to a ward.[12]

Ambulances transferred the injured with personal history cards attached to them to the evacuation hospital, located at a railhead. Nurses checked soldiers' records and sent some to the ward. A train or ambulance carried those needing more care to a base hospital.

Driving on shell-torn, muddy roads, ambulances swayed from side to side and noisy hospital trains jostled the passengers. Unfortunately the men endured unavoidable rough rides, long and painful.[12]

When Grace said, "the boys we got only had first aid," she meant that Base No. 17 admitted patients before they proceeded through

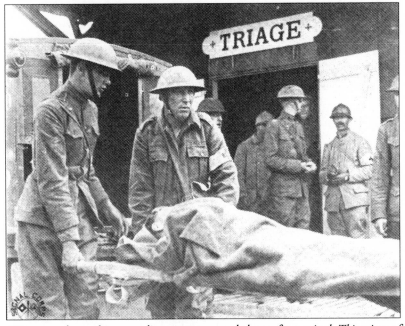

Triage sorted casualties according to urgency and chance for survival. This triage of the Forty-second Division was located near Suippes. (30)

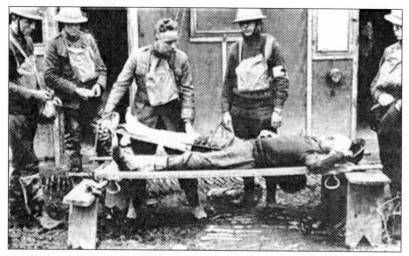

Medical personnel adjusted an improved splint on a litter patient in Broussey. (31)

the field, mobile, and evacuation hospital stages. In crisis times the Base No. 17 dealt with everything including triage and emergency surgery.

> Base Hospital No. 17 - Oct. 4, '18
> Dear Clarence,
>
> Your letter came today. I was so glad to hear from you; yours was the first letter I've had from the family.
>
> Am glad to hear you are coming right along in your work. It pays. And don't feel badly because you could not serve over here. You are doing just as much there. Will tell you lots of things when I get home that I can not write.
>
> I'm on night duty and working rather hard, especially when new convoys come in at night and night duty is hard anyway you know.
>
> The most wonderful vineyards in the world are said to be around here. We have seen the grape pickers at work and have seen them pressing the grapes for wine. You know how they do it, don't you? Get in the vat and stomp on them. Bare feet! Ugh! Spoiled my appetite for French wine.
>
> You know, the things you are likely to want to hear about,

are the things I can't write, but the papers are pretty nearly correct in what they say. I've read many things in the papers and then meet the people those things happened to, and the stories have always been straight.

Our boys are just as fine as can be. We love to take care of them. You tell Dad not to worry about me. I'm in the best of condition and very contented in my work. I tried to take some pictures of our quarters last week and a plain clothes man got after me. Told me I was liable for a court martial.

Everybody rides a bicycle here. Very few machines or horses. Bicycles are common as flies. So we rented some. Have to be in style you know. Had the time of our lives. My "bike" had peddles that would spin around without any regard for the wheels. Could go down hill but not up.

Will write every week and please do the same. Remember I'm pretty far away and that worrying business works both ways. Your letter was my first words in over two months. Sorry I can't tell you where I am but it is forbidden in the zone of advance. With my best love to you – from Grace

Grace's comment to Clarence, "don't feel badly because you could not serve over here," referred to her brother volunteering as a doctor in World War I. Because of his rheumatism, the army did not accept him. Proud of Clarence's contributions to medicine and the Mayo Clinic, she reassured him "you are doing just as much there." She wished Clarence could fulfill his desire to serve in France but she knew that wartime conditions presented too many health risks for him.

Every day Grace and other nurses put themselves in danger when they cared for sick doughboys, especially Spanish influenza cases. Since viruses were not yet discovered, the medical community failed to detect the cause of the disease. As a result, no effective vaccines for the flu existed. Physicians recommended wearing gauze face masks and quarantining for preventive measures. Nurses isolated flu patients and gave them the only known remedies, bed rest and

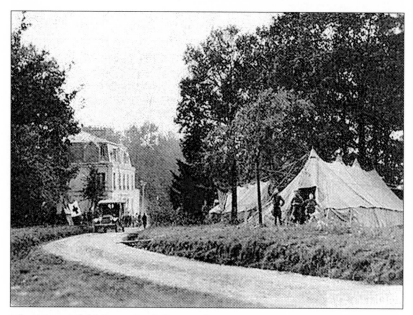

These tented field hospitals of the Fourth Division were set up at Chateau de la Foret.(32)

nourishment. They tried to protect them from complications such as pneumonia and meningitis.[13]

The peak and highly fatal months of the Spanish influenza pandemic spanned September through November 1918. During the same time period, over ninety-five thousand wounded from the Meuse-Argonne operation arrived at AEF hospitals and created a great demand for beds.[13]

Actually the 1918-1919 influenza did not originate in Spain. When eight million Spaniards contracted the flu, the neutral country had no censorship like the belligerent nations. When its newspapers reported the epidemic, people in other countries mistakenly assumed the disease came from Spain and, thus, the name.[13]

The deadly strain of influenza first broke out at Camp Funston (Fort Riley) in Kansas in March 1918 and spread to training camps nationwide. Hundreds and then thousands of soldiers got high fevers, disorientation, sore throats, back pain, headaches, and muscle cramps. The ill American troops embarked at U.S. ports and thousands became sick while crossing the Atlantic. After disembarking in Brest, hundreds died at Camp Pontanezen or in nearby AEF base hospitals.[13]

The Spanish influenza unleashed its fury somewhat simultaneously in Europe, Asia, and North America. During a twelve-month period, three unprecedented pandemic waves occurred in rapid succession with only brief intervals between them. From the spring of 1918 to the spring of 1919, the flu infected an estimated five hundred million, about one third of the world's population.[13]

Victims died within twelve to forty-eight hours after infection or later of secondary complications. Historically pandemics had claimed more lives of children and of adults over age sixty-five. However, during the 1918-1919 pandemic year, a unique phenomenon took place. Nearly half of the flu-related fatalities were young adults in their twenties and thirties.[13]

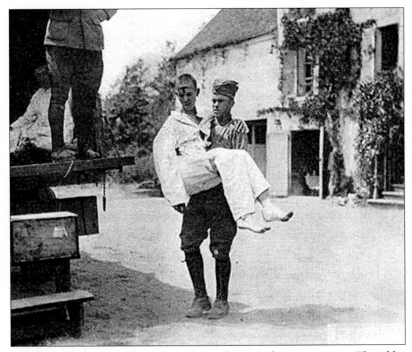

When necessary, army medical personnel carried patients during evacuation. This soldier was transported by truck from Field Hospital No. 15 near Montreuil. (33)

The disease killed an estimated fifty million people, and possibly as many as one hundred million. In comparison to the world's influenza deaths in one year, about ten million troops of all nations died in the Great War combat during four and a half years. Three hundred thousand American soldiers contracted the flu. The estimated number of U.S. troops who succumbed to the flu in 1918 ranges from twenty-three thousand to thirty-eight thousand. Eventually Spanish influenza caused the deaths of a half million Americans at home and abroad, almost ten times the over fifty-three thousand battle fatalities of doughboys.[13]

Grace's love for "our boys" motivated her to handle her demanding nursing schedule. She related her rare outings to her parents to persuade them not to worry.

Base Hospital No. 17 - Oct. 4, '18
Dear Mamma & Papa,

    I am doing night duty and we are very busy just now. The work is very very interesting. Our boys are the finest & best in the world. I love them all and am happy working for them. You never saw such patience and grit as they have.

    You know the Americans have their own trains here. I was surprised to find I could ride on a good old American train in France; as well as eat American food. We can have many things I did not expect to see. Of course we have our hardships, but don't think of us as actually suffering!

    France is very beautiful as you know. I love to get out of town into the country. One is always coming upon charming bits of country life, views, etc. And I'm learning to speak French. I will have lots of interesting things to tell you when I get home. It looks as if the war would not last much longer.

    Everything is very very expensive in France as well as in the U.S.A. France tempts one continually to spend money. Especially us women, even now in war times. I bought you a pretty bag, Mamma, a real "swell" one! Tho I hate that word swell. Stunning is better. Do write often. The mails are very slow. I'm writing once a week. My love to all who are interested. Tell them I'm well, interested in my work & happy. Much love, Grace

Grace rode on the American trains operated by the Services of Supply on standard-gauge and narrow-gauge tracks built by the Army Corps of Engineers. To support AEF wartime transportation needs, trains carried both freight and personnel. The Services of Supply imported 1,500 American locomotives and 18,000 freight cars in sections and then reassembled them in France. The engineers constructed rail yards and repair facilities.[14]

Base Hospital No. 17 - Oct. 16, '18
Dear Mamma & Papa,
 I haven't heard a word from you yet but I know you must have written. We are working hard but it looks as tho the end was in sight, doesn't it? The Boche is certainly running hard at present. One of the boys said, "I should say they are running. We can't keep up with them."
 France in war time is a different France than we saw when we were here before. What a difference there is between the old world and the new. And yet I'm enjoying it. I have some interesting pictures to show you when I get home.
 As usual, when I try to write a letter, I'd rather say too little than run a chance of doing harm or in any way giving the Germans an advantage. So, this lets you know I'm well and happy, and you do not need to be worried about me. My only trouble is a lack of mail. Do write often.
 Much love to all, Grace

After the officers and enlisted men of Base Hospital No. 115 started accepting patients in Vichy on September 11, the AEF gradually relieved the Base No. 115 nurses of their temporary assignments whenever possible. Grace and Edith received their orders on October 25, over two months after their arrival in Dijon. After

Grace's baptism-by-fire duty with stretcher cases and other casualties at Base No. 17, she knew what to expect in Vichy. She looked forward to rejoining her unit and using her valuable experiences at Dijon to aid many more doughboys at the hospital center.[15]

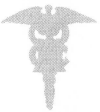

CHAPTER 5

Staying
After the Armistice

*It will be quite a long time before I will be home ... as long
as there are soldiers in France there must be hospitals.*[1]
—Grace Anderson

Hospital trains transported thousands of injured soldiers from
the Meuse-Argonne offensive, the final battle of World War I, over
three hundred miles to Vichy, a safe haven in peaceful countryside
on the Allier River.

The American Expeditionary Forces selected structures in the
historic resort and sites in other French spa towns for base hospitals. When Grace returned to Vichy, the base units had doubled to
four and treated troops in summer hotels, some formerly used as
hospitals by the French. The Army Corps of Engineers remodeled
the remaining hostelries to adapt to medical activities. By cluster-
ing about 75 percent of the base units into hospital centers in France,
the army economized on personnel, administration, and supplies.[2]

Grace reported to Base No. 115 in the nine-story Hotel Ruhl.
Base No. 1, Bellevue Hospital, New York City; No. 76, Camp
Greenleaf, Fort Oglethorpe, Georgia, and No. 19, Rochester, New
York, occupied an assortment of hotels. When No. 109 from Camp
Greenleaf arrived in November, the complex encompassed more

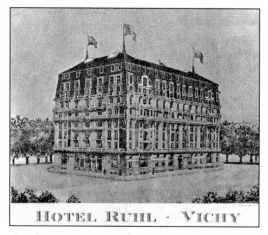

HOTEL RUHL · VICHY

Grace's unit, Base Hospital No. 115, occupied the Hotel Ruhl, shown in this sketch, at the Vichy Hospital Center. (34)

than sixty hotels and several additional buildings. The Vichy group, which had a normal bed capacity of 8,327, ranked as the fifth largest of the AEF's twenty-two hospital centers.[2,3]

Modern medicine practiced by the army contrasted with the cures of the nearby mineral springs, dating to the Greeks and Romans. In the 1860s Napoleon III made "taking the waters" for ailments fashionable. In the early twentieth century the affluent middle class reached Vichy by rail. During the Great War trains carried the wounded troops, rather than well-heeled travelers.

Usually hospital trains, mostly British, consisted of 360 beds and 16 coaches. The AEF designated cars for ordinary wards and specific purposes such as infectious diseases, pharmacy, kitchen, mess, and personnel. The staff included two medical officers, four nurses, three sergeants, two cooks, and thirty-one other enlisted men from the Medical Department.[4]

To relieve the forward facilities, a "pre-operative" train took some patients to base hospitals.

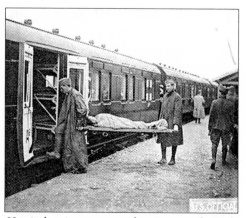

Hospital trains transported patients to the Vichy Hospital Center and other AEF medical facilities in France. (35)

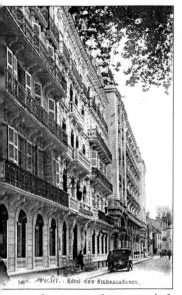

...ce sent her parents this postcard of Hotel des Ambassadeurs, used as ...arters for the nurses in Vichy. (36)

Before Base No. 109 joined them, nurses of the four base units totaled three hundred instead of the required four hundred. Those not yet in Vichy either awaited transportation or the AEF temporarily reassigned them closer to the front lines. The problem of an insufficient number of nurses persisted at the AEF centers.[5]

During the peak crisis at Vichy, Grace and her sister nurses cared for as many as twenty thousand patients fourteen or more hours a day. The Base No. 115 women accepted their demanding duties with ...n spirit. They highly regarded their chief nurse and command-...officer because, as Grace wrote, they "make everyone feel that ...y know the unit has honor and will do what is right."

At Vichy and all the centers, the chief nurse distributed the ...ses throughout the hospitals to meet the shifting needs of base ...ts. Grace worked mainly at Base No. 115 but also, when neces-..., at the other four hospitals.[5]

Vichy - Nov. 9, '18

Dear Clarence,

As you see by the heading, I'm back in Vichy and busy pouring ether. We are working very hard – no doubt about that, but it looks as if the war was over. I suppose you knew about the armistice a few hours after we did. You should see the French people. There were parades, and shouting and singing. I guess there will be some wildly exciting times if the Germans sign the armistice.

Only un-operated soldiers, whose conditions could t
and a ride of up to thirty-six hours, could be tra
special train.[4]

As carloads of injured troops arrived, the Vichy
the influx of new cases as expeditiously as possible
ether and gave fifty to sixty anesthetics, mostly lon
When she wrote her brother, Clarence, in Novemb(
being "really too tired to think, tonight, much less

> Vichy - Oct. 31, '18
> Dear Mamma & Papa,
>   I am back with my own unit, #115, again, an
> to be. We all think a great deal of our chief nurse
> the finest I have ever seen. We also admire the co
> head of the unit so you see some of the reasons we
> be back here.
>   They seem to always make things as pleasant :
> and everything goes with that spirit. Everyone worl
> and you know how much easier it is to work whe
> that way.
>   It looks as if the war was surely drawing to a clo
> be here for some time even so. It will be some t
> hospitals can be closed. I am giving anesthetics ;
> work is very heavy. I was beginning to feel pretty
> sitting down giving anesthetics is easier.
>   We are as comfortable as possible, in our qua
> They have turned one of the hotels into quarters for
> So except for not being quite warm enough, we are '
> antly situated. Write often. I think I have receive
> letters tho some were delayed. Much love to all, Gr

A photo of the five-story Hotel des Ambassadeur
a postcard Grace sent. She said: "Haven't we a fine I
where the nurses are living. There are three hundre
now."

I'm really too tired to think, tonight, much less write a letter but I just had to send you a line. We have very comfortable quarters. If we had a little more heat, and some hot water oftener we might almost imagine we were at home.

I shall stay over here as long as I can, even if peace is declared. Am perfectly happy here. I always have liked plenty of change you know. Am glad you are getting along as splendidly in your work. It's the only thing that lasts, that kind of success.

There are oceans of things I could tell you, I know, but they must wait. Have given between fifty and sixty anesthetics this week and most of them long ones. You know anesthetics are hard to give when you keep at them all day. Will try to write you once a week. Hope you'll do the same. With my best love, Grace

Because Clarence, her brother, encouraged her to learn anesthesia administration and helped train her, Grace served as an anesthetist earlier than most army nurses. Before U.S. entry in the war, American civilian nurse anesthetists went to Europe. Army nurse anesthetists belonged to base units, which opened hospitals in France during 1917. In January 1918 Grace began teaching anesthesia at Camp Pike. In April 1918 the army sent nurses to Mayo Clinic, where Grace observed anesthetists a year earlier.[6,7]

After nurses from Walter Reed General Hospital in Washington, D.C., participated in an intensive anesthetics course at Mayo Clinic, their hospital launched its own program. In early September several nurses from U.S. cantonments studied at Mayo Clinic. At their camps they instructed nurses, officers, and corpsmen.[7]

Later in September the acting surgeon general of the army directed commanding officers of hospitals in the U.S. and Europe to establish departments of anesthesia by training Army Nurse Corps personnel.[8]

At Vichy Grace proved her expertise in anesthetics, particularly the open-drop ether technique. She also administered nitrous oxide-oxygen anesthesia, which wartime surgeons found to be supe-

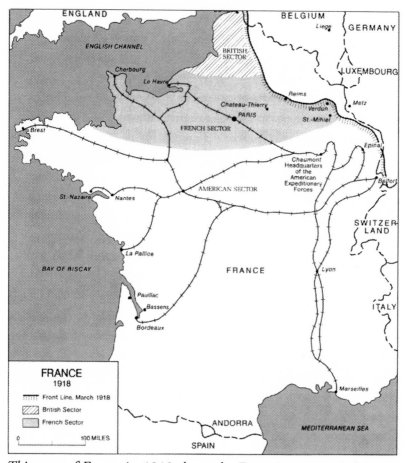

This map of France in 1918 shows the Front Line in March 1918, American Expeditionary Forces headquarters in Chaumont, American, British, and French Sectors, and the western ports of Brest, St. Nazaire, and Bordeaux.

rior to ether for gassed and shock cases.[9] Although she signed on as a regular nurse, her knowledge and experience earned her the Base No. 115 chief anesthetist position.

The army recognized Grace for her technical skills as well as her manner with patients. She calmed and reassured doughboys, especially those fighting anesthesia, to gain their trust and confidence. As a result, they followed her instructions on relaxing, inhaling, and exhaling.

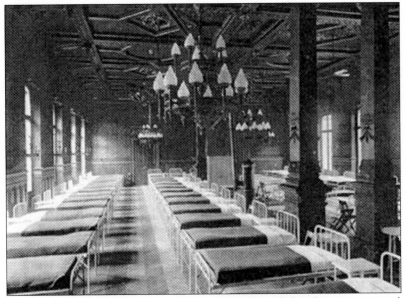

This ward of Base Hospital No. 1 in Vichy, photographed before the patients arrived, shows how the AEF transformed elegant summer hotels into hospitals (37)

Surgeons valued proficient anesthetists like Grace and she admired the surgical capabilities of the Medical Corps officers at Vichy. She developed good working relationships with surgeons, especially Capt. George Dillard Wells. George, from Base No. 76, was a civilian surgeon for seven years in Missouri. Grace and George had much in common because they both were born and educated in middle America and grew up in large families.

Proud of Clarence and his success in the Mayo Clinic roentgenology department, she shared his news about the study and use of X-rays with George and other surgeons. Since physicians relied on X-ray technology to identify battlefield injuries, the Army Medical Department had a roentgenological service consisting of medical officers, knowledgeable in X-ray work, officer-technicians, and enlisted men. An X-ray course in the United States and additional instruction in France at the Bazoilles Hospital Center school supplemented the officers' previous experience.[10]

Evacuation, mobile, and fixed field hospitals X-rayed 80 percent to 95 percent of the patients. The AEF utilized portable bedside units rather than full-size X-ray machines, unsuitable for the French current. The doctors closer to the front briefly described fractures, located any foreign bodies, and recorded evidence in chest wounds. As a result, surgeons seldom requested X-rays during an operation. Base hospitals also used portable X-ray machines, especially for troops who came directly from the front.[10]

Vichy - Nov. 12, '18
Dear Clarence,

You are so faithful about writing regularly to me, and it means so much to get letters over here. They must have torn the country to pieces over there when peace was declared (or rather armistice signed). They tried to here but you know the French don't know how to really "rough house."

This is a funny country in many ways but very fascinating to me. The art in everything appeals so strongly, the landscapes even seem planned to make a picture wherever you look. The painstaking way they do everything is almost ridiculous sometimes, as for instance, our operating room gowns. They are of French make with deep pleats from a yoke to the hem and every time they are laundered the pleats are pressed in. Imagine!

Our convalescent officers are quartered in the old home of the Countess Sevigne who was the friend of Napoleon. It is a most charming place; and until you have seen France you don't know the meaning of the word charming. The gardens are wonderful.

In the park in front of our hospital (the Hotel Ruhl), is an old stone pillar, which was placed there by Caesar at the time of the invasion of Gaul. Did I tell you that the Hotel Ruhl is the place where the Kaiser headquartered when he used to visit Vichy? And the proprietor of the hotel was a German sympathizer of course. So when war was declared and he shouted "Long live Germany," his guests rushed him to the roof of the hotel and threw him off; so I'm told.

Wish you were here to enjoy France with me; but you will come someday under pleasanter conditions, when traveling is a pleasure and not a trial. Our traveling has had to be done chiefly at night; sometimes with no lights for fear of air raids, sometimes packed in like sardines, all except once, without being able to lie down. But once, – our last journey – was on the "At-a-boy" special, the American train, and we had berths and got up to a real breakfast on a diner! Imagine the U.S. even building railroads over here.

Some country we have, Son.

Heaps of love, Grace

Vichy - Nov. 14, '18

Dear Mamma & Papa,

The war is over, as you all know, by this time. It will be quite a long time before I will be home, tho, as it will take a long time to evacuate all these hospitals and even when the wounded are sent back to the States, as long as there are soldiers in France there must be hospitals. Vichy will be one of the permanent hospital centers.

We are very busy. I give anesthetics all day long, which is very hard work. It is getting cold but the weather is very nice here in Vichy. So much nicer than in Dijon where it rained all the time.

It was wonderful to be here at the finish of the war. We had the news nearly twenty four hours before you did. At eleven o'clock that day of the armistice signing the bells began ringing, guns firing and people shouting, everybody wildly happy. Then an American bugler blew "taps." It seemed so appropriate. That "go to sleep, go to sleep;" peace! The war is over!

That night there was a parade, the wildest thing imaginable. The parade and the crowd got so mixed up you couldn't tell which was one & which the other. And they ran, jumped, hopped, yelled; it certainly was wild. Old men and old women, little children, soldiers, civilians all mixed together.

It is beautiful weather, but there is so little heat in the buildings that at this minute I have on two suits of underwear & two sweaters and a bathrobe over all. That sounds like forty below zero, and it isn't at all. If the houses were warm we'd think it quite mild out. But you have to pile on the clothes.

I shall not try to send Xmas things as they are so apt to get lost. I'll bring some things home when I come. Everything is very expensive so we can't get many things anyway. Candy we simply can't buy. Fruit is very expensive; melons cost about seventy-five cents apiece when bought in large quantities for our mess even. Pears are about thirty cents apiece, apples a dollar a dozen. I think butter is something like $1.50 a lb. This is no time nor place to save money, you see. Much love to all, Grace

The armistice news spread with lightning speed from London and Paris to the towns and villages of Europe. Spontaneous festivities like the one Grace saw in Vichy broke out in the Allies' countries. Some soldiers, both Americans and Allies, marched in impromptu parades. Other men were too exhausted and battle-stressed to celebrate.[11]

When the news crossed the Atlantic to the United States, rollicking citizens crowded outside the White House in Washington and filled New York's Times Square. In Chicago celebrants covered their heads with wastebaskets to avoid the objects that jubilant people tossed into the air.[11]

People around the world danced in the streets. They also felt weary and grieved the loss of millions of loved ones in the Great War. Soon Americans turned from revelry to the country's rallying cry, "bring the boys back home."[11]

Vichy - Dec. 6, '18

My dearest Brother! —

Your most generous gift arrived today — was brought directly to me in the operating room. Was not expecting any kind of a Christmas gift, but as usual, in some manner, you divined that a leave was in sight, and sent a gift that will come in mighty handy, I can tell you!

Now Miss Muir and I (we are still together) will go to Nice right after Xmas. If we can make Paris too, we will; and of course we are going up to Chateau Thierry.

You know I never was sent directly to the front, but we were in the zone of advance. Our hospital was 80 miles from the lines. We worked harder there than they did at the front because we worked steady all the time and at the front they had a let up when there wasn't a drive on.

And the boys we got, had only had "first aid" you know, when they came to us. Our convoys always came in at night, so the day forces had to stay up & help take care of the arrivals. The last convoy we got before I left that hospital were all stretcher cases and such a sight I never want to see again.

Our work now is with drainage cases chiefly and amputations of limbs they have tried to save and find it impossible to do so. I would be very happy here if I didn't have so much heartache for these boys of ours. They are the best ever; their spirit is wonderful. But to see so many cripples and mutilations; the worst of all are the jaw cases, I think. Have you seen any of those cases with the lower jaw gone entirely? It is so pathetic. They are doing some wonderful plastics and the dentists are doing a lot with jaws.

It has rather amused me to be put in as chief anesthetist over the nurses who signed up as the unit anesthetists. As you know I didn't mention it, but went in as a regular nurse.

I'm wearing more clothes than I ever wore at once in my life before. One reason is the lack of heat in the buildings. Most of the time we get in bed to keep warm when off duty, or else go out doors and exercise. Our rooms are very nice; full of great big plate glass mirrors and marble fireplaces, like all French houses are, and we have French beds that are really luxurious after the cots we had in Dijon. Those cots were tent shaped at the center. Our heads hung one way & our feet the other.

We have a bathroom off our room and sometimes we have hot water. When the water is hot everyone is very excited, and there is a great scramble for baths. The first one is lucky. She gets a fairly warm bath. The next one hangs over the faucet watching to see how long it lasts and finds by the time she has drawn six inches it is icy cold again.

Damn is a very common word over here and very popular. It is beginning to slip off our tongues very gracefully. Six inches of water body temperature in a warm room, could pass if you had nothing more; but try it some time in an icy cold bathroom.

Then our steam radiator. We used to embrace it fondly every time we entered the room and remark how comfy it would make us in cold weather. That was before we had been properly introduced to French steam radiators. Now it gets a kick or a knock every time any one gets near it. It's never been more than lukewarm. Now don't get the idea that we are really suffering, for we are not. Uncle Sam wouldn't let us really suffer. Our mess is still good.

We have a chief nurse & commanding officer who are the best ever. They both treat us all like we were their own families. Never nag, never spy around, but make everyone feel that they know the unit has honor and will do what is right.

Last night at dinner, some French beggars or street musicians came into our dining room to play for us, (not by request I can assure you). They chose the middle of the meal, when everyone was cramming in food so as to hustle back on duty, to play the Star Spangled Banner. It was dreadfully funny to see everyone standing at attention with their mouths full of food.

It was great to be here when the armistice was signed. Would love to be in Paris now during the peace conference, but no chance. You can't get rooms for love or money and besides the A.E.F. is ordered to stay away. Shall make a try.

We have very little flu here now. I never did have it but most of the nurses did. Several died. Two died here at Vichy and the same day had a double funeral.

Thank you again, Dear, you are very kind and thoughtful. With oceans of love and best Christmas wishes, Grace

P.S. Some patriotic boy to sell your car and walk! Am somewhat worried about your rheumatism. Take care of yourself and let me hear how you are.

In her December 6 letter Grace mentioned that nurses she knew contracted the Spanish flu. Her two friends at Vichy, who succumbed to the flu, were among the over two hundred deaths (236 to 268 by some estimates) of Army Nurse Corps members in the United States and overseas. Influenza and pneumonia caused most of the deaths. Others died as a result of ship, airplane, train, and automobile accidents but none from enemy action.[12]

Grace's comment to Clarence about the "amputations of limbs they have tried to save and find it impossible to do so" indicated how hard surgeons worked to keep soldiers whole. Seeing so many "cripples and mutilations" upset Grace who had "so much heartache for these boys of ours."

The Vichy center received severe and complicated cases that had crushed limbs, deeply embedded shell fragments, and complex head, face, and jaw injuries requiring extensive treatment. As they pro-

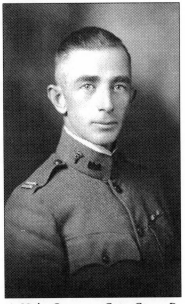

At Vichy Grace met Capt. George D. Wells, U.S. Army Medical Corps, a surgeon with Base Hospital No. 76. (38)

gressed through the casualty handling stages, those men endured emergency surgeries, initial procedures such as probing for fragments and the cutting of dead tissue. Although stabilized, their agony did not stop.

During crisis times mangled and maimed troops kept tables in the operating rooms busy day and night. Critical surgeries took an emotional toll on the medical personnel. Grace felt more comfortable talking to her friend, George, than any other surgeons about their common challenges.

Grace and George supported one another in their ongoing personal struggle to balance professional detachment and concentration on the surgery with an awareness that the "case" was someone's son. Major war injuries brought daily ups and downs to the surgical team. They shifted between satisfaction when doughboys survived life-threatening wounds to emptiness when their best efforts failed to save a life or limbs.

As Grace wrote Clarence, "the worst of all are the jaw cases, I think. Have you seen any of those cases with the lower jaw gone entirely? It is so pathetic." In World War I surgeons operated on more jaws in a few months than they did in years at civilian hospitals. By gaining expertise in those operations, surgeons reflected the medical profession's growing emphasis on specialization to ensure the most effective treatment.[13]

Grace pointed out "they are doing some wonderful plastics and the dentists are doing a lot with jaws." Since the AEF designated Base No. 115 to care for jaw and face injuries, Grace frequently administered anesthetics to those patients. She saw first hand how maxillofacial surgeons in cooperation with dental surgeons, who were assigned prosthetics and splints, helped the difficult and "pathetic" cases.[13]

Base No. 115, equipped with some oral and plastic instruments and emergency jaw splints, lacked supplies and materials because of delayed shipments. The medical staff ingeniously produced makeshift solutions for the pressing needs to offer specialized care. The maxillofacial patients also benefited from the talents of highly skilled modelers in wax reproductions. The sculptors shaped facial parts and surgeons tried to transform soldiers' disfigurements into their pre-war appearance.[13]

The Vichy center housed the art department of the Army Medical Museum in Washington, D.C. An army expert in anatomical art supervised prominent U.S. artists and sculptors who traveled to the AEF hospital centers. They made historical drawings and castes of special cases for future surgical use. The art department sent over two thousand drawings, photographs, and masks to the museum in Washington, D.C.[13,14]

Grace's chief anesthetist job involved her in a wide variety of surgeries, especially those related to the head. The Vichy hospitals developed a reputation in the AEF as being the principal facilities for all head injuries. Since Base No. 115 received the majority of head cases, Grace gave anesthetics to many of those troops. Although the soldiers wore steel helmets, head injuries accounted for an estimated 16 percent of all wounds. Doctors attempted to improve the grim statistic that more than 50 percent of the penetrating skull wounds became fatal.[13]

Grace worked with ophthalmology teams as they treated contagious infections and wounds of eyelids and orbits. When eyes could not be saved, the AEF optical unit in Paris supplied artificial eyes. The Vichy center and those in Paris and Savenay trained the blind before transporting the men home.[13]

The army credited the Base No. 115 neurologists and neurosurgeons for making a successful start in establishing a district neurological center. Grace served alongside neurosurgeons who finished the surgery for doughboys passed on to them from the advance section. During rush periods at the front, time constraints and the need to handle as many cases as possible hindered surgeons from completing tedious head and peripheral nerve operations. They temporarily prevented the destruction of nerves by extensive debridement before sending patients requiring additional surgery to Vichy.[13]

The AEF hospitals welcomed the periodic visits of distinguished U.S. physicians and surgeons recruited by the army as senior consultants. Among them was Col. George W. Crile, Medical Corps, who had conceptualized the base hospital system. Dr. Crile served as senior consultant in surgical research. Medical officers in France sought the advice of those leaders in general medicine, surgery, and various specialties.[15]

Vichy - Dec. 18, '18
Dear Mother,

Received your letter written the 21st of November today. Have been receiving your letters alright, now. You see they have had to follow me around and so were slow in reaching me until now.

Guess I wrote you about the celebrations here when the armistice was signed, but I don't think that the celebrations here were nearly as great as in the States. Old world people are too slow going. However, at heart they are even more thankful, as indeed, they have cause to be.

We have many rumors of going home soon but nobody knows anything. I was not anxious to go home till I heard Clarence was sick and now they can't send me any too soon. If he is going to need care I'm the one to be on the job, and I won't let anyone else have my job if I can help it!

I'm very worried, Mother. Please write me often, every few days at least, every day if you can, and let me know how he is. I was going to ask for a transfer and stay over here for a year or so but now I won't. I'll come home soon as I can. You do not need to worry about me. Physically I'm very well but I certainly am worried about Clarence.

Am going to Nice for a few days and to Paris, right after Christmas. I do need a little change but not because I'm working hard or am not well! Am unusually well. Also the work is getting very light, and besides I have an assistant.

Oceans of love to you all, from Grace

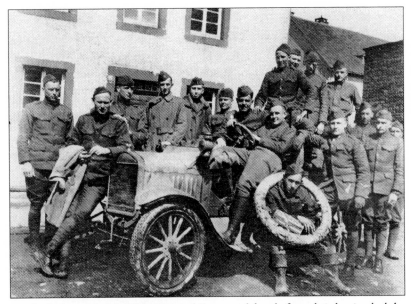

Medical personnel at the Vichy Hospital Center took breaks from their hectic schedules. Capt. George Wells is fourth from left behind the Model T. (39)

Grace's workload started to lighten because thirty-eight base units journeyed to France in November and December.[16] When the American forces began conducting operations on a large scale in the summer of 1918, the existing number of base hospitals proved inadequate and stayed that way until the armistice. During the Great War the shipping schedule allowed hospital units in proportion of four to a division. However, combat troops often displaced medical personnel and equipment.[17]

Hundreds of urgently needed nurses still waited for space on transports. After the war ended in November, 1,500 nurses arrived in France.[18] The total of Army Nurse Corps members in the AEF reached 10,245 and army nurses at home and abroad peaked at 21,480.[19]

In the post-armistice days Grace, Edith, George, and other friends socialized more frequently. The Red Cross paid for recreation huts and coordinated events. Chaplains organized morale-boosting sports, motion pictures, shows, music, and dances.[20]

Actors and musicians sailed to Europe to perform for the doughboys. Talented staff and patients also entertained. Base units even formed bands and the Red Cross furnished the instruments.[20] The officers at Vichy enjoyed a unique club, a rococo casino once frequented by princes and industrial barons.[21]

When humorous incidents occurred during recreation hours they appeared as tidbits in the social columns of *The Caduceus.* The popular Vichy center newspaper primarily reported important AEF activities.[22]

Vichy - Dec. 18, '18

Dear Clarence,

Mother's letter saying you are at home, just came. Seeing that you are a man of leisure for awhile I'm going to write often, maybe everyday, for awhile.

Isn't that an awful threat? That's what you get for being under the weather. Now lad, do be sensible and loaf, for a long time. Hope you won't have to stay in bed long, but better a little too long than not long enough.

Well, it rains today. Yes, today, tomorrow and the next day. When the sun peeps out of gray clouds – everyone says "Oh see the sun," – and it is gone again! But it is nice. France is lovely; I love it. I don't want to be French but I'm glad to be an American in France.

Have changed French teachers. My little refugee is going back to her home in Nancy, (and that is near the border, you know,) so I must get a new teacher. And my new teacher is an American. She is an old lady, seventy years I should judge, but very interesting. An old singer who came here first to study. It is slow learning to talk it seems, but now is my time and I'm trying to make the most of it.

We have a great many ex-prisoners here. They say if it had not been for the American Red Cross they would have starved. German bread given them was made with sawdust. They say when they dropped it the sawdust would fall out on the floor.

When they got their first Red Cross boxes they say they were like children. They sat & hugged their boxes 12 hours at a time afraid to go to sleep for fear of losing them. But they have been taken care of by the Red Cross for four or five months and look pretty good tho they all have that queer color all prisoners have.

Shall enclose this with Mother's letter. Take good care of yourself. Is there anything you would like to have from over here? If there is, let me know & I'll try to get it for you. With my love, Grace

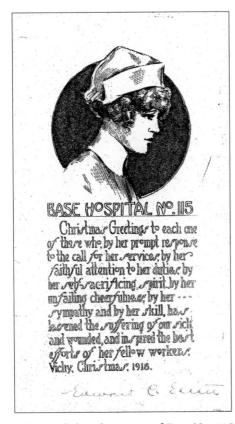

Grace celebrated 1918 Christmas at a Red Cross party that featured a living pictures presentation. The depictions included the old masters such as *Madonna and Child* by Giovanni Bellini to modern art like *The Sunshine Girl* by Raphael Kirchner.[23]

Lt. Col. Edward C. Ellett, M.C., commanding officer of Base No. 115, gave Grace and the other women in her unit the Christmas gift of a personal message accompanied by the drawing of a World War I nurse.[23]

"Christmas Greetings to each one of those who by her prompt response to the call for her services, by her faithful attention to her duties, by her self-sacrificing

Grace and the other nurses of Base No. 115 received the drawing of a World War I nurse with a message from their commanding officer as a Christmas gift. (40)

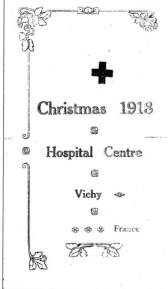

The Red Cross hosted the 1918 Christmas party at the Vichy Hospital Center. (41)

spirit, by her unfailing cheerfulness, by her sympathy and by her skill, has lessened the suffering of our sick and wounded, and inspired the best efforts of her fellow workers." [23]

After more than four months of long days and weeks at Dijon and Vichy, the AEF granted leaves to Grace and Edith. Grace looked forward to reporting her travels to Clarence, to cheer him up and encourage him to sail to Europe in the future.

As Grace and George socialized at holiday events, their friendship grew stronger but remained professional. However, they unexpectedly became romantically attracted to one another. The situation troubled Grace since she had proper relationships with several other married doctors. She realized they were teetering on a dangerous brink and had to step back and regain their balance. She and George welcomed her leave to put distance between them. They promised to get back on the right course when Grace returned.

CHAPTER 6

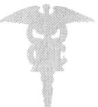

Making
Postwar Decisions

It is hard to be over here and know there are sick ones in the family ... I feel I'm needed more at home than here now.[1]
—Grace Anderson

Throngs of travelers crisscrossed France during January 1919, two months after World War I ended. The United States demobilization effort transported 125,356 troops across the Atlantic in late 1918. The AEF continued processing soldiers by the hundreds of thousands at the western ports of Brest, St. Nazaire, and Bordeaux.[2]

The doughboys, exhausted and grimy from months of trench warfare, cleaned up and rested at embarkation camps. After lining up for physical exams, records inspection, and payroll, the men anxiously awaited their voyage. Delays in departures dashed hopes for a speedy return.[2]

The U.S. government lacked many of the Allied ships that carried Americans to France and struggled to comply with the public's demand of "bring the boys back home." In response to the pleas, the United States scheduled enough transports for 115,382 troops in January and planned a steady increase in upcoming months.[2]

While soldiers headed to the west coast of France, Grace and Edith journeyed south. They joined crowds of military personnel and French civilians who squeezed into trains for post-armistice trips. Grace reported on her sightseeing to persuade Clarence to visit Europe with her in the future.

Nice, France - Jan. 7, '19
Dear Clarence,

As you see by the heading, I am on the Riviera for a rest. It is very interesting as you can imagine, but not purely French like the towns in the north; therefore, not so quaint. This is the season – the hotels are crowded. Our rooms overlook the park; palm trees and flowers, and beyond, the great sweeping view of the Mediterranean.

It is raining today. The weather is very changeable so we hope for sunshine tomorrow. We are going by automobile to Monte Carlo and Menton, which is on the Italian border. We are only allowed to go three miles over the border however. Another trip we are planning, will take us to Grasse, and we will visit the grotto.

We enjoyed our stay at Marseilles. I think every nationality in the world is there. You probably know it is the wickedest city in the world. There are portions of the city which no American is allowed to visit. It is so bad it is beyond one's imagination to picture it.

In the harbor is the island you have read about in The Count of Monte Cristo – you remember the Chateau d'If where he was imprisoned and escaped by jumping into the sea, or allowing himself to be thrown in for a dead man. It looks like brigand country. It is easy to believe such things happened here.

Traveling is very difficult now. The crowds are so great that if we didn't always meet some fine American man we would have a hard time. We are always taken care of by our men. The Americans are the finest in the world and they just simply accomplish what seems impossible. We women all feel we are surrounded by protectors all the time. Hope you are feeling better. Do write. Oceans of love, Grace

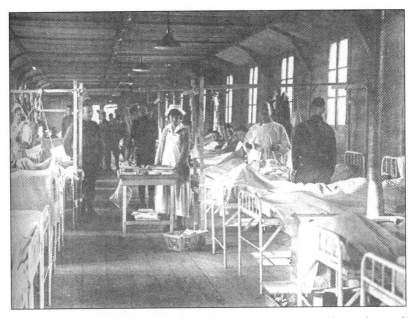

This surgical ward at Allerey Hospital Center in France was similar to the wards where Grace's operating room patients recovered at Vichy. (42)

Vichy - Jan. 14, '19

Dear Mamma,

I just came back from my leave of absence and found your letter written the fourteenth of December. I feel so badly about being over here and everyone working so hard at home. I wish I could get back to take care of Clarence.

Just how serious is his sickness? Who is his doctor and what does he say about his condition? I'm worried to death, of course, so be sure to tell me the truth.

I just got word that the girl I roomed with all thru training, Eileen Forrest, died over here in France. It is an awful shock to me. I thought a lot of her. I hope Marian & Kenneth are better. It is hard to be over here and know there are sick ones in the family at home.

I shall write the news I have to tell to Clarence and you can read his letter. This is to ask you how he is and to tell you how sorry I am that I can not be there helping you. I shall ask to be transferred home immediately but I do not know if I will get it.

I shall write Clarence tomorrow. I have written often. I don't see why you don't get all my letters. Tell Papa that card is great. I have it hung on my wall already. Heaps of love to you all and hoping to see you soon, Grace

Vichy - Jan. 15, '19
Dear Brother Clarence,

Just returned from my leave and must tell of all the interesting cities I saw. The first place we stopped going south was Marseilles. It lies, as you know, among the mountains along the coast. The views from the heights are wonderful and I'm sending you some views.

We saw Gaby De Lys play here. Marseilles is her home city. She has a beautiful home here. This is a great city for flowers and in one act she, (Gaby) throws baskets of violets to the audience. The play lasted three hours, was very spectacular and very splendid in spite of the fact that it was French and hard to understand, (and too long!).

Traveling is very hard and very expensive – such crowds on the trains, in hotels, etc., but you can get excellent meals and it sure tasted good after army fare.

Nice is interesting in a different way, being more of a resort. Fine hotels all along the waterfront, & casinos, etc. Of course we went to Monte Carlo. Didn't waste any of our hard earned francs there tho. The gambling rooms are beautiful and they do a rushing business all the year around. Persons in uniform are allowed in the place from 9 to 10 a.m. After that the gambling begins. The casino lies just above the water and is surrounded by gardens with statuary, etc. The oranges are ripe on the trees there now. Palm trees, oranges & flowers look good to Minnesotans in January.

We visited Menton and from there went over the border

into Italy. Had several trips into the mountains, the maritime Alps. Going home, we crossed the "Basses Alps" or low Alps going to Digne, Grenoble & Lyons.

So we went from flowers to snow. Saw Mont Blanc from Grenoble, but were not allowed to go into Switzerland. Was surprised to find the weather on the Riviera very much like Minnesota fall weather. Quite a little snap in it. It is necessary to dress warmly. Winter clothes are the thing and not straw hats and sun shades, as I used to imagine.

Hope you are much better by the time you get this letter. Am trying to come home as soon as possible. Wish I could have been with you all thru your sickness. Am putting in for a discharge as I feel I'm needed more at home than here now.

Can't tell you how badly I feel cause you are sick. But you are a good sport, Laddie. I won't go so far away again. I do want to be at home taking care of you.

With my best love, and hoping to be with you before so very long, Grace

After Grace wrote to her mother and Clarence, she continued worrying about her brother and the slow mail delivery from France to the United States. She cabled an urgent message to her parents the same day.

WESTERN UNION CABLEGRAM
29 NA JD CABLE VICHY JAN 15 1919
A.F. ANDERSON REDWING, MINN.
CABLE IF BROTHER NEEDS ME
WILL GET DISCHARGE.
GRACE ANDERSON 654PM

The next day Grace watched for a cable and inquired about an emergency army discharge. On January 17, she received sad news in a letter dated December 29 from Ella, her cousin.

Vichy - Jan. 17, '19

Dear Mamma & Papa,

Have just heard of Clarence's death. I feel heart-broken. My dear dear brother. I can't write much now. I hope to be home soon.

There is talk of the unit going back to the states in a month or so. If it doesn't I shall ask for a discharge. I am very well. Do not be worried about me in any way.

Am so sorry I went into the service but it seemed the thing for me to do at the time. The world seems very empty to me without my brother. There is one thing I am thankful for, he was at home and not over here among strangers as he might have been. If I could only have taken care of him.

Do not worry about me as we will cable if anything happens. I have very good friends with me and our chief nurse is like a mother to us all. It has all been a terrible strain on you both. May our God comfort you and keep you safe till I return.

With my dearest love, Grace

Worried about her brother, Clarence, Grace sent this cablegram to her parents in Red Wing, Minnesota. (43)

Clarence's death devastated Grace, especially since she wrote him letters after he had passed away on December 28. She wished her family had cabled her in mid-December when her brother's condition worsened. However, she knew they understood the difficulties of World War I transportation. The Atlantic crossing and train ride to Minnesota took over two weeks. Arranging an army discharge and obtaining space on a troopship could add a month or even more.

Grace regretted staying in the army when Clarence became ill in November. She agonized about not being home to care for her brother in his last days. Aware that her grieving could affect her demanding anesthesia work, she changed to night nursing for awhile. Honoring Clarence, she carried on with her "duties to the living."

Vichy - Jan. 19, '19

Dear Mamma & Papa,

Just a note again today. I can't write much without giving way too much to my grief, and I have duties to the living; it won't do to depress them with my sorrow.

Please keep every record of Clarence you can for me. Everything, the newspaper accounts and all. I want some for my very own, to keep. Oh, I love him so much I can't bear to think of him being gone. Did he leave a goodbye for me?

Sometime I'll tell you how he came to me in a dream early one morning the later part of December. I can't write it now. Please send me word of him soon. I haven't heard from the family, only Cousin Ella's letter. Did he suffer much? Oh, mother, how can we live without him? He has written me such wonderful letters since I have been away, he was such a wonderful brother to me. His last letter to me brought his Christmas gift.

I think of you, too, mother, and of Papa, and know how hard it is for you and how hard it has been. And I way over here not able to help my own when they need me. If we could only look ahead. If I could only have known.

Do write soon or if it is too hard, have Arthur [her brother] do it for you. I hope to be home in a couple of months. I can't get there any sooner than that, I don't think.

I cabled a few days ago. I hadn't heard anything and was so worried. The next day I got Cousin Ella's letter. I shall try to write every day from now on. I hope you don't worry about me. I am well and conditions are fine here. Very little sickness now and the work getting very light.

If anything should happen you would know at once as my friend who has been with me all the time since I entered the service, is still rooming with me & will cable. But nothing is likely to happen so do not be worried. You have had so much to go thru I don't want to add to your troubles.

I am longing to be home again, and hope the time will pass quickly till we sail. Ella's letter written the 29th of Dec. reached me Jan. 17th. With all my love, Grace

When Grace's mother mailed her "the newspaper accounts and all," she learned about Clarence's sickness and death. Complications of rheumatism or a rheumatic disease unknown in 1918 forced Clarence to leave his Mayo Clinic position as assistant in the roentgenology department in mid-November. Clarence and his colleagues tried various medicines and treatments but to no avail. His illness progressed to the critical and then terminal stage.

Clarence mentioned Grace often and insisted that she stay in France rather than make the long trip to Red Wing. He thought it was more important for his sister to care for the injured doughboys. Grace, the Andersons, and numerous people loved and admired Clarence for always putting his concern for others before himself. So her brother's unselfish request in his final hours did not surprise her. Realizing she had done what Clarence wanted her to do, eased her sorrow. Proud of her brother's achievements, Grace appreciated the tribute to him in the *Red Wing Daily Republican.*

The obituary, "Death Calls Dr. C. W. Anderson - Skilled Physician and Surgeon of Mayo Clinic," pointed out that Clarence, at

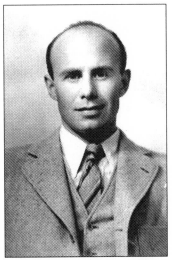

Dr. Clarence Anderson, Grace's brother, passed away in December 1918 at age 32. (14)

the age of thirty-two, was "one of the prominent young physicians and surgeons of the Northwest." He served as the assistant chief surgeon at the Illinois Central Railway Hospital in Paducah, Kentucky, a year after he received his medical degree from Louisville Medical College in 1911. He also "established a fine practice in Hudson, Wyoming" before returning to Minnesota.

"Dr. Anderson's skill as a surgeon and physician was recognized and in a few months he became associated with the Mayo Clinic where he remained ... until his health began to fail him ... Dr. Anderson was of a splendid type of young man. He was highly successful in his surgical career and he acquired many friends, who will be grieved to learn of his passing."[3]

Clarence never met two of his "many friends," Edith and George, who felt they knew him well because Grace spoke about her brother frequently. They comforted Grace and encouraged her to talk about Clarence as a way to cope with her loss.

During two weeks of night duty, Grace gave full attention to her patients. When off-duty she lifted her spirits by socializing with Edith and George and sharing stories about Clarence. Soon everybody would be leaving Vichy.

Following the armistice, the Army Medical Department started demobilization. The AEF canceled orders for future hospitals, stopped most construction work underway but completed some structures. Base units gradually transferred troops who had recovered enough for the voyage home and reduced the number of beds by 50 percent, wherever possible. Eventually new cases no longer arrived.[4]

During January fifty-one units, mostly those that reached France in 1917 and by the summer of 1918, ceased to function. Two of them, Bases No. 1 and No. 19 in Vichy, prepared to close their hospitals by January 20. The patient load at Vichy had decreased from a peak of twenty thousand to only one thousand.[5]

The hospitals shipped back to the United States certain medical property, such as surgical instruments and equipment for X-ray and scientific laboratories. Since the Vichy units occupied French buildings, they needed to pack supplies and equipment for removal and storage in a medical supply depot. Each hospital sent a final sick and wounded report to the AEF chief surgeon.[4,5]

Grace, Edith, George, and everyone at Vichy attended farewell parties for the first two groups of medical personnel with departure orders.

Vichy - Jan. 23, '19

Dear Mamma & Papa,

We received notice (official) that our unit will be leaving Vichy about the middle of March. We expect that means we will go to the states.

Nurses are being asked to volunteer to stay over here as they say they are still badly needed, but I do not feel that I can stay. By the time we go home I will have been in the service a year and a half and I guess that will have to be my "bit."

I am well but not happy since the sad news of Clarence's illness and death. Of course I think a lot about it all, and I think after all if I had not come into the service he might have, because he wrote me that he saw a way of getting into the service after all, when I was at Camp Pike.

I wrote and talked him out of it. At least he stopped talking about it, when he heard about conditions. So maybe it was best so. It was hard on me to be so far away, but if that prevented him from being away, and meeting death among strangers and perhaps without good care and the comfort of your presence, that is much to be thankful for.

I am worried now for fear the strain on you both has been too great & you will be ill. There is no reason for you to be at all worried about me as conditions here are good.

Write as often as you can till the first of March. After that, cable if anything happens, as letters would not reach me. Your last letter came to me in 17 days. Isn't that excellent time? Much love to all, Grace

On January 29, *The Caduceus,* the center newspaper, published a front-page story, "Vichy Hospital Center Will Be Abandoned As Speedily As Possible. Statue of Liberty Will Be Reality Soon For All Yanks in Vichy." When asked how long it would take to clear Vichy of Yanks, Col. Walter D. Webb, commanding officer, said: "At the end of two months there won't be a Yank in Vichy, with possibly the exception of M.P. and R.T.O. men."[6]

Vichy - Jan. 30, '19
Dear Mamma,

Just a line tonight. We will leave for the states about the time you get this letter unless there is some delay. I am well but very anxious to get home. I shall not write much, tonight, because there isn't much new happening now.

I asked for a change from the operating rooms and have been on night duty for two weeks. I go back to the operating room tomorrow. There isn't much to do. There are only a thousand patients in the whole center now and some more will leave for the states tomorrow. That is quite different from the twenty thousand we had here a few months ago, or even weeks ago. Much love to you all, Grace

When Grace resumed administering anesthesia in the operating rooms, she and George saw each other more often. Their special bond, created by sharing life and death surgery situations, grew stronger. The sudden passing of Clarence, and Grace's dependence on George, drew them even closer.

As base unit friends exchanged goodbyes, Grace and George became caught up in the emotions sweeping through the center. They no longer could deny their love for one another. Their passion overtook propriety and turned their friendship into a romantic relationship.

Their clandestine liaison, out of character for both of them, conflicted with their personal morality and the social mores. As a refined woman, Grace conformed to high standards. She regretted straying from her values and shirking the responsibility given to the women of her era. American society expected her to be a guardian of moral conduct for herself and also for men.[7] Grace's head told her that she must douse the flames of romance, but the decision tore at her heart.

Vichy - Feb. 6, '19

Dear Mamma & Papa,

I have just been asked to go up into Germany with the army of occupation & have consented to go. I had to decide in five minutes and it seems the thing for me to do.

I wanted to go home & had all my plans made but this will delay it for a short time. If our boys need us we have got to stay a little longer. Hope it won't be more than a couple of months.

Will send you my new address as soon as I can. We are going to Coblenz, Germany. Write me often as you can and cable me if anything is wrong at home. I will get a discharge & return to the U.S.A. as quickly as possible in case you need me. You can cable me at my expense.

I'll send you a signed check and you can fill in the amount. If I'm sure you will cable me I will be able to keep from worrying so much, so promise me. Hope you are well. I have not heard from you for a couple of weeks. I expect to leave Vichy tomorrow night.

With all my love, Grace

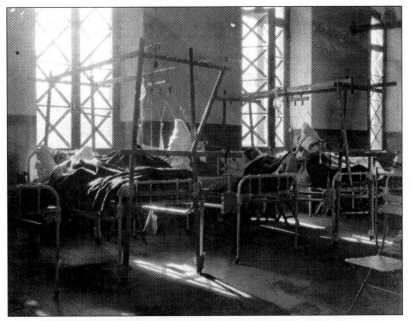

*Grace took this photo of her patients in the fracture ward
at Vichy Hospital Center. (44)*

In Germany, Grace planned to immerse herself in nursing duties rather than dwell on her problems. By helping the soldiers recover, she believed her heartaches of losing Clarence and ending her romance with George would heal in time.

Before going their separate ways, Grace and George promised to remain good friends and to keep in touch. On February 7, five days before Base Hospital No. 115 closed, Grace traveled by rail to Coblenz, Germany.[8] On February 14, two weeks after his Base Hospital No. 76 ceased to function, George entrained for Neufchateau, France, where he reported to the advance section headquarters for his next orders.[9]

American Army of Occupation, 1918

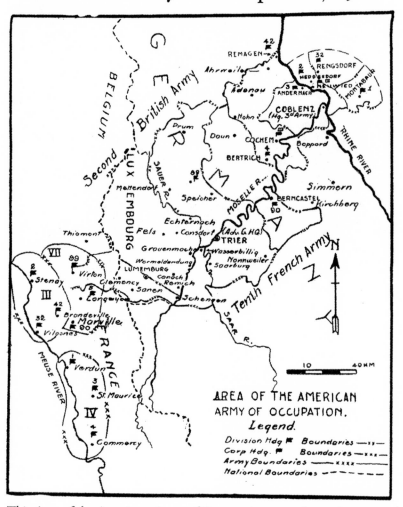

This Area of the American Army of Occupation map shows the assigned territory in Germany, which stretched from the borders of Luxembourg to the Rhine River, and had only two large towns, Coblenz and Trier.

CHAPTER 7

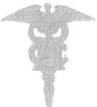

Aiding the
Army of Occupation

*If our boys need us, we have got
to stay a little longer.*[1]
—Grace Anderson

The bombardment of bursting artillery shells, explosions of aerial torpedoes, and the firing of machine guns and rifles devastated a village and a forest near Chateau-Thierry on the Marne River. Seven months afterward, Grace visited the battlefield where cataclysm left eerie silence and stark images in its wake. Ruins, rubble, and twisted trees spread across the land where horrific combat waged during June 1918.[2]

The Americans proved their capabilities and determination to the Allies and the Germans at Chateau-Thierry. The American Expeditionary Forces suffered heavy casualties including over one thousand men in the Marine Brigade, killed and injured on one calamitous day, June 6. In spite of their losses in the battle, the heroic marines drove through the dark forest of Belleau Wood and held their positions to thwart the German advance to Paris.[2]

Grace, among the thousands who traveled to the battlefields after the Great War, paid her respects to the Americans who made the ultimate sacrifice. She honored "our boys" in rugged cemeteries

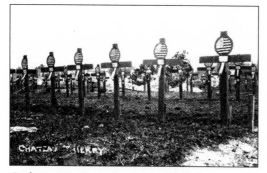

On her way to Germany, Grace visited the cemeteries in the Chateau-Thierry area. (45)

where rows of crosses marked the graves decorated with flags and wreaths.[3]

Following her sobering trip to the war's western front, Grace turned her attention to the Third Army, organized as the army of occupation. When she reached her destination in February 1919, the maximum number of troops sent by the United States to Germany was located in the historic Moselle River Valley. A total of 262,259 U.S. soldiers occupied the assigned territory stretching from the Luxemburg borders to the Rhine River. About one million people resided in the region that had only two large towns, Treves (Trier) and Coblenz.[4]

The army billeted Grace in the home of a German doctor in Coblenz. "They treated us fine," she wrote. " I think they are afraid to do otherwise." While in Coblenz Grace and her nurse friends discovered the army restricted some sightseeing. They obtained permission from the U.S. military police headquarters detachment to enter Schloss Stolzenfels castle on a hillside overlooking the Rhine River. The police stamped the seal of the provost marshal, Third Army, AEF, on an official memorandum to the palace guards.[5]

Grace reported to Evacuation Hospital No. 26 on February 13 and settled into the nurses' quarters in a nearby Neuenahr hotel. She found that evacuation hospitals functioned as

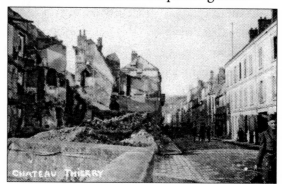

Grace saw the war ruins at Chateau-Thierry. (46)

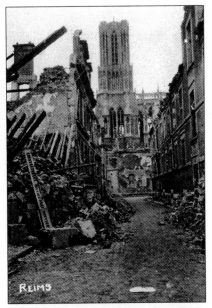

While touring the World War I battlefields, Grace purchased photos of the destruction in Reims and other French locations. (47)

fully equipped base hospitals like her previous duty stations in France. The staffs worked in buildings constructed for hospital use as well as in schools and military barracks.[6]

The army grouped hospitals in centers, as much as possible, to develop special services. In Coblenz, at the largest center, each of the five evacuation hospitals admitted certain kinds of cases such as surgical, orthopedic, medical, and neuropsychiatric.[7]

The Third Army's extensive area required a few isolated hospitals at outlying points. After the 1918 march into Germany, the army selected a site at Neuenahr, in the extreme left of the American sector, for a hospital to serve the Forty-second Division (The Rainbow Division).[6,7]

Hospital No. 26, formerly a spacious hotel, provided two thousand beds, half of those in former schools. The hospital transferred fracture and mental cases to Coblenz but handled convalescent and all other patients.[6,7] Since war casualties no longer filled the hospitals, surgeries decreased. As a result, Grace primarily cared for troops with influenza and pneumonia rather than administer anesthesia.

Neuenahr, Germany - Feb. 14, '19

Dear Mamma & Papa,

As you see, I'm up in Germany with the army of occupation. We like it the best of any place we have been yet. Have fine places to live and fine hospitals. We were billeted with a German doctor's family in Coblenz for a couple of days & they treated us fine. I think they are afraid to do otherwise.

This is much more comfortable country to live in than France. We have some snow and quite cold weather, but our houses are warmer. I spent a few days in Paris, a short time in Metz, have been up thru the battle front at Chateau Thierry and Toul, and a couple of days at Coblenz.

The Americans actually rule the country up here. It did me good yesterday when our soldiers were standing at "Retreat" and the Star Spangled Banner was played, to see the Germans stop and take off their hats to our flag.

The Germans treat us Americans wonderfully well. I suspect that is German propaganda. We are at a very beautiful town, and famous German resort. They have hot springs here, it is a health resort, also. We are north of Coblenz and south of Cologne, on the western side of the Rhine and about four miles inland. I shall write you often, and I still have hopes of being home this summer. Write me often as you can. With much love to you all, from Grace

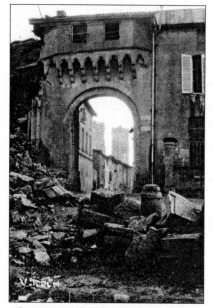

The constant bombardment during the Battle of Verdun in 1916 caused almost one million casualties. (48)

Grace's Metz postcard reflected how the French reacted when they recovered the city, under German rule since 1871. Photos, before and after World War I, showed a German Kaiser statue standing atop a Metz monument and then lying on the ground. Grace said, "This is the statue you have read about at Metz that was torn down. A French soldier was put where the Kaiser statue was."

Grace correctly suspected "Germans treat us Americans wonderfully well" for propaganda purposes. When U.S.

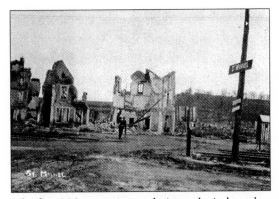

The first U.S. operation and victory by independent American-led forces occurred at St. Mihiel, southeast of Verdun. (49)

soldiers paraded through the streets of Coblenz, Germans warmly welcomed them. Apparently defeated German commanders instructed civic leaders to persuade their citizens to hide any bitterness. Officials hoped a friendly appearance would produce more favorable terms for Germany at the peace conference in Versailles.[8]

Neuenahr, Germany - Feb. 28, '19

Dear Mamma & Papa,

Am still in Germany, and will be here for a couple of months more, I think, but you know you can't tell anything about the army.

We have excellent food and I guess I told you we are living in German hotels. They just tell the Germans to get out and they go, and in move the Americans. They must hate us but they treat us very well.

The apollinaris water springs are here. The bottling works must cover about thirty city blocks. The Americans have turned part of it into a bakery. The Americans have turned the park into a stable yard or horse yard and one place I saw our horses stabled in a big porch. These things seem kind of tough but it is only giving them a little taste of their own medicine. There are hot sulfur springs here and everyone is taking the baths.

We live very quietly here with many restrictions. One nurse is not allowed on the street alone even in the daytime; and at night there must be at least two nurses & an officer. We are with the third army of occupation and the Rainbow Division.

You asked about my wool quilt, Mamma, some time ago I meant to tell you I have it with me and don't know what I would have done without it. We have had to sleep in cold rooms and with not enough blankets sometimes and then the air is so damp over here in winter the wool is the only thing to keep you warm.

We still have influenza and pneumonia here, but I don't believe it is as bad as in the states. These boys are getting excellent care. Better care than patients get in civilian hospitals at home. We have plenty of food and bedding and everything to work with and a beautiful hospital.

I was surprised to hear of Harry Crosse's [family friend] marriage but lots of boys are marrying French girls. How do his people like it I wonder. I think there will be lots of homesick French girls in the U.S.A. after the war. Much love, Grace

The U.S. government created the Forty-second Division in August 1917 by combining National Guard units from twenty-six states and the District of Columbia. Col. Douglas MacArthur, the

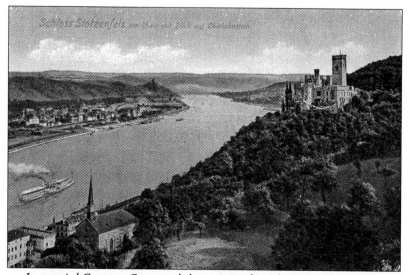

*In occupied Germany Grace needed permission from the U.S. military police
to tour the Schloss Stolzenfels castle overlooking the Rhine River. (50)*

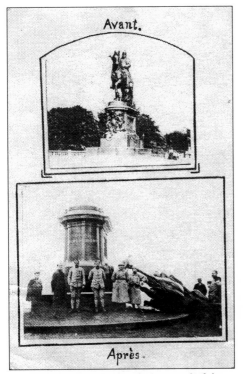

Avant.

Après.

Grace sent her parents this postcard of the toppled German Kaiser statue in Metz. (51)

new division's chief of staff (later its commander), remarked: "The 42nd Division stretches like a Rainbow from one end of America to the other." The Rainbow Division, among the first American divisions on the western front, became part of the Third Army in Germany.[9]

From mid-February to mid-March, Grace got acquainted with occupied Germany and adjusted to her schedule at Neuenahr. George attended patients in France at Camp Hospital No. 9 in Chateau Villain, and then at the Base Hospital Center in Mesves.

The nine Mesves hospitals claimed fame as the largest AEF center for having a daily capacity of twenty-five thousand beds during the November 11 to December 5, 1918 period.[10]

Neuenahr, Germany - Mar. 3, '19
Dear Mamma,

I have been talking with a young German girl this morning and thought you might be interested to know what she said about prices of things over here.

She says for soap, she has to pay 12 marks a bar for laundry soap, 8 marks for soap like ivory, & 8 marks for toilet soap. An ordinary nice bath towel she says she has to pay 60 marks for, and she said for bed sheets of very poor quality – almost like cheese cloth, 80 marks. A mark is worth about 16 or 17 cents now. She wanted to buy my old shoes that I consider about ready to throw away for 40 marks.

It makes you feel sorry for these poor women over here. This girl's sister is getting ready to be married and she begged me to sell her my bath towel, so her sister could have two, she has one already.

When I told her what we were paid by our government & how our clothes were furnished she asked me to take her back with me to America. My, I really felt sorry for her. They really are hard put to it, and all for that villain Kaiser.

Of course I'm not wasting too much sympathy on these old "dyed in the wool" Germans. But when you see these children of the poor come to the door begging for food, and, when given a couple slices of bread, carefully stow it away in the bag on their backs to carry home, it kind of grips your heart; for we Americans have never seen much of that before.

There are many wealthy looking people on the streets too, and they look fat and healthy, but the poorer classes are having a time of it. This girl says they do not expect much relief for the next two years. She is only about twenty years old, and she is coming to me to learn English.

At the same time I'm learning German, not because I like the language but I like to keep my ears open and understand what they are saying around here. You know I studied German in school so I have a foundation.

How is it with you people? Is it still hard to get things? Is food very high now? I think food is cheaper now in France than in the U.S. And clothes I know are cheaper in France. If I could afford it I would buy some embroidered table linen to take home, it is so beautiful in France and such wonderful old linen but it takes twenty-five dollars or more apiece so I guess I won't.

Well, I am enclosing a check for twenty-five dollars. Please buy some flowers for me for Clarence's grave for Easter and Memorial Day. What you have left is for you. I'm also sending a blank check. If you need anything for yourself you can use it. I should have a couple of hundred in the bank. With much love, Grace

Grace empathized with the poor people. Many were starving because the war ruined the country's food production. The Allies continued a naval blockage until Germany signed the final peace treaty so the Germans could not obtain food elsewhere. Since Germany depended on imported products and raw materials, the shortage of supplies drove up the prices of consumer goods.[11]

The young German woman, who begged Grace to sell her a bath towel and well-worn shoes, epitomized the poorer population. The government added taxes onto the cost of goods, resulting in the poor paying a larger proportion of their income than the rich. The animosity between classes grew during the war and lasted after the armistice. The "wealthy-looking" residents, who Grace noticed on the streets, enjoyed a comfortable lifestyle. Fellow Germans begged for food and clothing while hoping for relief.[11]

The American Red Cross provided food, shelter, and free medical care to the refugees in Germany. The Red Cross transported sick children to hospitals, established orphanages, and found relatives for the elderly. The U.S. Food Administration, under the leadership of Herbert Hoover, saved refugees from starvation and aided their survival with the basic necessities.[11]

A month after Grace arrived in Germany, the last unit in Vichy, Base No. 109, ceased to function March 12. The hospital center

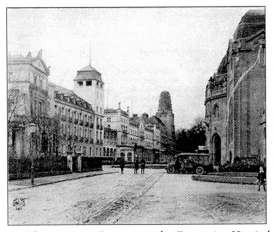

In February 1919 Grace reported to Evacuation Hospital No. 26 in Neuenahr, Germany. (52)

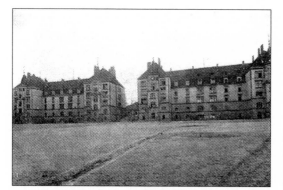

Hospital No. 26, where Grace worked, transferred some patients to these surgical and medical wards of the Coblenz Hospital Center.(53)

opened April 9, 1918 and cared for over forty-six thousand patients during its year of activity.[12] Only six of the fifty-one hospital units, which closed in January, departed that same month or in February. The remaining units waited until March and April when they, and a half million doughboys, sailed back to the United States.[13]

Important events occurred in Grace's life in the days between her March 3 and March 31 letters. On March 18, George came to Coblenz with an army detachment from France. While awaiting further orders, he visited Grace in Neuenahr. Less than two months after they parted, they faced a new and unexpected challenge. Grace's doctor confirmed her pregnancy.

The news stunned them and drew them back together in an even more complex relationship, but still a platonic one, as they had decided in Vichy. As Grace and George processed what was happening in their lives, they discussed their options.

They both agreed with the anti-abortion laws, in effect in all the states, and believed abortion was immoral. They knew that unwed pregnancy and single parenting carried social stigma. The U.S. society regarded single mothers as fallen women who lacked obedience to authority and sexual restraint. Maternity homes, a refuge for unwed mothers, offered adoption, as did agencies. But Grace wanted to keep the baby rather than pursue the more socially acceptable option.[14]

George never considered divorce because they ended their romance in Vichy. Neither of them had seen divorce, although not rare in 1919,[14] among friends or family members. They realized that divorce caused difficulties for everyone involved, especially the children, like George's five-year-old daughter.

The army's standards of social conduct presented another concern. In France the army was unaware of their offenses against the moral code. Nevertheless, they were contrite about conflicting with personal morals.

They worried about the Army Nurse Corps, which viewed out-of-wedlock pregnancy as misconduct. In World War I the ANC treated its pregnant nurses leniently. However, those women endured the humiliation of being relieved from active service and sent home in disgrace.[15] If Grace suffered the same fate, George no longer could monitor her health. The separation and the distance would prevent future discussions of their situation. As a result, they carefully guarded their secret, known only to her trusted doctor in Neuenahr. Grace, of course, never disclosed her emotional turmoil in her correspondence.

Neuenahr, Germany - Mar. 31, '19
Dear Mamma,

Your letter of March 5th came today and I surely was glad to get it. Yes I am very anxious to go home and think surely I will be there soon. I think it is just as well that I didn't leave for home during the bad weather because I got a little run down and would have probably been sick on the way. I felt so bad about Clarence that I lost weight. If I had been traveling it might have meant pneumonia or something serious.

Am glad Margaret & Nell [her sisters-in-law] are so good to you. Mamma you can't know how much I want to get home. We are allowed to take short trips around the country to places of interest but I have not gone anywhere. Am going to take care of myself till the weather settles. It has been very raw, damp and cold.

No Mamma dear, I do not need a single thing. Uncle Sam and the American Red Cross take good care of us all. They will furnish us everything we need down to tooth brushes & tooth paste even. We surely cannot complain of anything except a lack of heat.

And money, no, I do not need any. I've spent nearly all I've made over here but I'm never in the hole, and am very comfortable. Tell Papa that I appreciate his thoughtfulness in letting me know how money affairs are going to be for me in the future. It is of course a big comfort to have something back of me for old age!

I hope your dividends are good so you can have every comfort possible always. Don't think of us children first, think of yourselves. Tomorrow I will be thirty-five years old. I will be middle aged before I know it, time goes so fast.

Am glad Wells Jr. [her nephew] is home again, but his experiences were probably good for him. The revolutions, etc., we don't see anything of here in the Rhine valley. We just read the papers as you do. The Germans here are very well behaved and respectful.

I didn't get this finished last night and here it is April first and a beautiful bright clear day. I am going out for a walk when I have finished this letter. We have had so much cold damp snowy rainy weather we are happy when we see a bright day.

Papa would enjoy a trip on the Rhine at this time, when he would see the American patrol boats going up and down, stopping and inspecting the German boats as they please. It is some sight to see the Stars and Stripes on the Rhine. Much love to all but especially to you and Papa, from Grace

From the end of March to mid-May, George was stationed southwest of Coblenz and Neuenahr. His assignment with Ambulance Company No. 155 of the Seventh Corps Sanitary Train allowed him to communicate regularly with Grace and see her occasionally. After the armistice the Seventh Corps became a part of the Third Army and set up headquarters at Wittlich in the western portion of the American sector.[16]

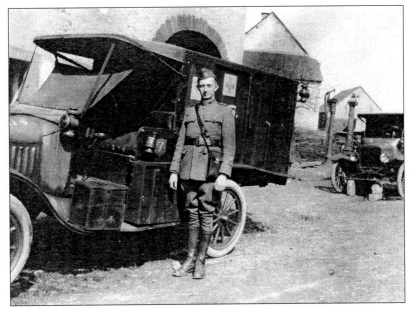

Capt. George D. Wells assumed command of Ambulance Co. 155,
Seventh Corps Sanitary Train, in Wittich, Germany. (54)

The ambulance companies evacuated and aided thousands of casualties in the midst of World War I military operations. Ambulance companies serving the Third Army operated from central points in Treves (Trier) and Coblenz. They provided ambulances for evacuation hospitals in those cities and answered calls from local and remote places for transportation of sick or injured troops. The companies also loaded hospital trains for evacuations from the area of occupation.[16]

In early April George adapted to his new responsibilities and Grace cared for her patients. When she suddenly felt ill, Grace attributed her sickness to her pregnancy. She continued working until symptoms of the Spanish influenza alarmed her. Her doctor hospitalized her immediately.

Having seen soldiers and nurses die from the flu, Grace feared for her baby and herself. Her parents might lose two children in less than a year as well as an unborn grandchild. She summoned all her strength to survive the disease.

After consulting the physicians at the Coblenz center, George and Grace's doctor gave her an optimistic prognosis. They assured her that her influenza appeared lighter than most cases during the height of the pandemic. They concurred with the physicians at Coblenz who believed the Spanish flu had run its course.[17]

The news boosted Grace's determination to get well. During the next two weeks George contacted her doctor and followed her progress. Although weakened, she improved enough to write her mother a note.

Neuenahr, Germany - Apr. 13, '19
Dear Mamma,

I hope to be home this summer. Am almost sure I will be. Everything is very quiet here. We have some very sick boys but not very many.

I got my birthday card yesterday. Many thanks. This is a great month for anniversaries, my birthday, Papa's birthday, your wedding anniversary & Fred's [her brother] anniversary. I'll be thinking of you all on those days, and am sending my congratulations. Much love to all, Grace

On April 15, 1919, George assumed command of Ambulance Company No. 155. During the war each of the eighty-two evacuation ambulance companies used twenty or more ambulances. After the armistice, when the companies became available to hospital centers, each had twelve ambulances. The personnel included one Medical Corps officer and thirty-nine enlisted men.[18]

George checked on Grace as she gradually recovered and resumed her nursing duties. Grace's April 24 letter to her parents reflected a change in her attitude. Undoubtedly, the gamut of emotions she experienced while in Europe overwhelmed her.

Neuenahr, Germany - Apr. 24 '19
Dear Mamma & Papa,

Still up in Germany, and very much fed up with it. We are

not busy now and time hangs heavy on our hands. I shall try to get a discharge soon, but maybe it will be turned down. Shall try tho.

It is still damp and rainy here with plenty of chill in the air. We have a little stove in our room and it feels very good to have a fire. You don't know how it will seem to us all to get home. In the army you can't move hardly without permission and after a year and a half of it, it is getting awfully tiresome.

There isn't much to write about and I don't feel like writing today so this is only a word to let you know I'm well. Tomorrow is Papa's birthday. Hope it will be a happy one. And today is your wedding anniversary. Many happy returns of both holidays. With best love, Grace

Soon after Grace mailed her letter, she received an official memo of appreciation to the AEF women from Gen. John J. Pershing, commander-in-chief of the American Expeditionary Forces.

France, April 30, 1919 – General Orders No. 73
TO THE WOMEN MEMBERS OF THE A.E.F.

While the achievements of American Arms are still fresh in our memories, I desire to express my sincere appreciation of the work done by the women of the American Expeditionary Forces. The part played by women in winning the war has been an important one. Whether ministering to the sick and wounded or engaged in the innumerable activities requiring aid, the cheerfulness, loyalty and efficiency which have characterized your efforts deserve the highest praise. You have added new laurels to the already splendid record of American womanhood.

It is a privilege to testify that your glorious accomplishments in the war have given you a new place in the hearts of officers and men of the Army, and have earned for you the admiration of a grateful nation.
JOHN J. PERSHING
General, Commander in Chief [19]

General Pershing's praise lifted Grace out of the doldrums. Right before Mother's Day her doctor pronounced Grace and her baby healthy after the difficult first three months. Adding to her elation, the army notified the nurses that Hospital No. 26 might close soon.

Neuenahr, Germany - May 12, '19

Dear Mamma,

This is Sunday, Mother's Day, and everyone is writing home. They have tried to make it a pleasant day for us. We had a fine dinner and a yellow rose at each place. We had roast beef, mashed potatoes, cauliflower with egg, jam, pickles, fruit salad, apple pie and ice cream.

But best of all is the report that we are to leave here for home next Wednesday. We have asked to go but did not expect it so soon. We are not sure it is true but if you do not hear from me again soon you can think of me as on the way home.

I may be delayed after reaching New York, but at least you will know that I am on that side of the water as I will write you from New York. I may have to have a loan of some money when I get there if I can't draw mine from the bank, but will telegraph if I need it. It is sometimes slow getting your pay from the government.

The weather is warm at last but the Red Wing boy who said a month ago that we were having weather "like June in Minnesota," must be warm blooded as we have had to have fires, wear wool dresses and sweaters until the last two days. I still am wearing my winter underwear, but then it has taken me a long time to get over the flu.

By the way, you didn't know I had it, did you? I was in the hospital but I am getting fat now, and haven't felt so well for a long time. The hospital work is very light now. Think they will let everyone go home who wishes to. Don't expect me till you see me but things look very bright.

Much love to you all, Grace

In May of 1919 the size of the Third Army decreased. Hospital No. 26 in Neuenahr and four other evacuation hospitals in Coblenz, Treves (Trier), and Prum transferred special services to the remaining facilities. Army nurses served with the American forces until they departed Germany in 1923.[20]

As Grace planned her long journey back to U.S. soil, she and George remained in a quandary about their future relationship. They agreed to make decisions regarding their complicated lives when they both returned to the United States. At the same time George wrote the AEF chief surgeon and asked for hospital duty because it

(FOR OFFICIAL CIRCULATION ONLY)   (G.O.73)

G. H. Q.
AMERICAN EXPEDITIONARY FORCES,

General Orders)   France, April 30, 1919.
NO. 73   )

TO THE WOMAN MEMBERS OF THE A.E.F.

While the achievements of American Arms are still fresh in our memories, I desire to express my sincere appreciation of the work done by the women of the American Expeditionary Forces. The part played by women in winning the war has been an important one. Whether ministering to the sick and wounded or engaged in the innumerable activities requiring aid, the cheerfulness, loyalty and efficiency which have characterized your efforts deserve the highest praise. You have added new laurels to the already splendid record of American womanhood.

It is a privilege to testify that your glorious accomplishments in the war have given you a new place in the hearts of officers and men of the Army, and have earned for you the admiration of a grateful nation.

JOHN J. PERSHING
General, Commander in Chief.

Official:
ROBERT C.DAVIS,
Adjutant General.

A True Copy

W.F.Toevons
2nd Lieut.,S.C.,U.S.A.

Gen. John J. Pershing, commander-in-chief of the American Expeditionary Forces, sent this letter to the women of the AEF. (55)

better suited his previous military and civilian surgery experience. In another memo to the commanding general, Seventh Army Corps, George requested his first leave since his overseas duty began in September 1918.[21]

Grace entrained in Germany and arrived at the Headquarters Hospital Center in Vannes, France, on May 18.[22] While Grace awaited her departure orders, she took a short leave in late May to see George. He traveled to France to check on Grace's health, to get details of her embarkation, and inquire about a possible hospital assignment. In Vannes, as in Vichy, they went their separate ways once again. For the first time since they met they would live an ocean apart.

Grace proceeded to the Kerhuen Hospital Center in Brest on June 1. Eight days later she embarked on the *New Amsterdam*.[22] She no longer dreaded attacks by submarines or wearing the Red Cross rubber suit with weighted feet to keep her upright in the water. Instead, other uncertainties loomed on the horizon. During the voyage she prepared how she would stay afloat in the rough seas of social stigma until her life could reach a safe harbor.

CHAPTER 8

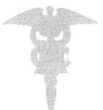

Returning
to America

Please wire me a hundred dollars at once. Our pay is
held up ... Am well. Hope to be home soon.[1]
—Grace Anderson

The ships carrying American troops streamed into New York
harbor from November 1918 through June 1919 and afterward,
either as a trickle or a torrent, depending on available transports.[2]
Unlike the secretive departures during wartime, tugs and fireboats
greeted the vessels. On shore people waved flags and sang as a band
played patriotic music.

The crowd cheered Grace and all the passengers as they disembarked from the *New Amsterdam* and headed for demobilization
camps or stations. Grace was among 364,183 Americans who arrived in June, the month with the greatest number of returnees.[2]

The United States successfully transported 1,623,251 across the
Atlantic in only eight months. Other survivors of the Great War
included hospital patients rotated home before the armistice and
soldiers in Germany for occupation duty.[2]

Grace addressed a Department for Reception of Returning
Troops postcard to her parents. She filled in her name, date, unit,

and ship. "Well Done Men - America Greets You," a Statue of Liberty photo, and the YMCA logo appeared on the postcard.[3]

The staff at the nurses' station in the Hotel Albert notified Grace of her future World War I premium, "to be covered by personal remittance," and her "per diem allowance of a flat rate of $4.00 for 2 days, paid in advance."[4] The delay of her pay prompted a telegram, the one she mentioned in her last letter from Germany.

NEW YORK, NY JUNE 21, 1919
A F ANDERSON
712 BUSH ST RED WING MINN
PLEASE WIRE ME A HUNDRED DOLLARS AT ONCE
OUR PAY IS HELD UP AND AM BROKE MY MONEY
WILL BE SENT HOME TO ME LATER AM WELL
HOPE TO BE HOME SOON
GRACE ANDERSON, HOTEL ALBERT,
NEW YORK CITY

In New York Grace caught up on national news, especially about Congress passing the Nineteenth Amendment on June 4. Women throughout the country were celebrating their right-to-vote victory following an over seventy-year struggle for suffrage. Grace, her sister nurses, and all American women, who participated in the war effort, had more reasons to rejoice. The U.S. government acknowledged that their patriotic contributions at home and abroad proved their capabilities and also advanced the suffrage cause.[5]

In January 1918, while Grace trained at Camp Pike, President Woodrow Wilson endorsed the Nineteenth Amendment. The House of Representatives narrowly approved it but the Senate refused to debate the amendment until October. At Hotel Albert Grace learned how the final act of the Washington drama unfolded with glacial speed.[5]

After a nine-month delay and a plea from Wilson, the Senate defeated the bill by two votes in October 1918, and then by only one vote in February 1919. When the last session of the Sixty-fifth

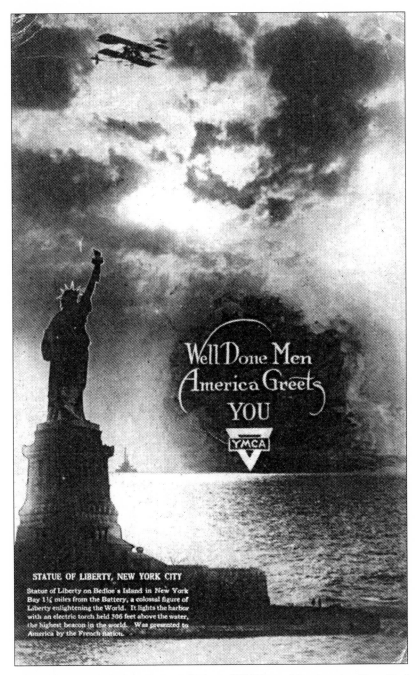

STATUE OF LIBERTY, NEW YORK CITY

Statue of Liberty on Bedloe's Island in New York Bay 1¾ miles from the Battery, a colossal figure of Liberty enlightening the World. It lights the harbor with an electric torch held 306 feet above the water, the highest beacon in the world. Was presented to America by the French nation.

The Andersons received this Statue of Liberty "Well Done Men America Greets You"
postcard when Grace returned from Europe.(56)

Congress ended, suffragists complained about waiting until the new Congress started for another vote. Suffragist leaders redoubled their efforts to gain the required two-thirds majority for the bill. The National American Woman Suffrage Association emphasized their patriotic wartime activities while trying to persuade Wilson and Congress to do more for the suffrage cause. The National Woman's Party picketed the White House again.[5]

Wilson called the Sixty-sixth Congress into a special session in May 1919 and repeated his previous endorsement. Finally both the House and Senate passed the Nineteenth Amendment and sent it to the forty-eight states for ratification by thirty-six states or three-fourths majority. New York and eight other states ratified in June.[5]

Grace and other nurses hoped for a quick approval. They also wished the government would recognize their war service by giving them relative rank. Nurses held only a paramilitary status during World War I. They fulfilled demanding responsibilities without the rank or benefits they deserved. The Army Nurse Corps continued lobbying aggressively. To the delight of Grace and all army nurses, the ANC campaign started picking up speed when nursing organizations and women's associations and colleges rallied with the corps.[6]

Grace completed demobilization at Hotel Albert and then took steps to combat the stigma of her pregnancy. Knowing she faced an uphill climb, Grace set a safer course for herself. She contacted friends from her Base No. 115 and Base No. 1, a Vichy Hospital Center unit organized at Bellevue Hospital in Manhattan. She asked for help in finding a job and living quarters, far from the glare of her small hometown in the Midwest.

About the same time that Grace reached the United States, George began an assignment at Camp Hospital No. 33 in Pontanezen, France. Hospital No. 33 served the largest AEF camp and the entire port of Brest. Pontanezen provided the reception area for most U.S. troops. After the armistice, doughboys rested there prior to boarding vessels.[7]

Hospital No. 33 opened in January 1918 in an old French concrete barracks and expanded to a three-story modern building, extra barracks, and forty more structures. By June 1919, when George joined the staff, the hospital had admitted more than twenty-eight thousand patients.[7] George adjusted to his new surgery duties in Europe and, in the meantime, Grace went to Minnesota. Her military record stated:

"Left this station June 26, 1919 to proceed to her home for relief from active duty in the military service at the expiration of accrued leave due per Par. 74 SO 171 Hg. Pt. of Emb. Hoboken, N.J. dated June 20, 1919. Final payment to include to Aug. 10, 1919 and bonus by check No. 8936 for $208.83.

"With the approval of the Secretary of War and by order of the Surgeon General the reserve nurse within named is relieved from active duty in the military establishment to take effect Aug. 10, 1919."[8]

As Grace approached Red Wing on the train, she anticipated a bittersweet reunion. Her secret of nearly five months would shock her parents. Like other families of World War I soldiers, the Andersons expected Grace to be the same as the day she joined the army.

Driven by patriotism, Grace devoted a year and a half to her country in a realm of critical medical decisions. In her letters she purposely shielded her family from any unpleasant details of wartime nursing.

The Andersons were overjoyed and grateful to see Grace alive, well, and on U.S. soil. However, her romance and out-of-wedlock pregnancy stunned her parents, both pillars of their local Methodist church and the community. They loved their daughter but disapproved of her indiscretions.

Grace wanted to spend several months in Red Wing but staying a long time undoubtedly would trigger a scandal. To protect her well-respected mother and father from any humiliation, she purchased a round-trip ticket. She arranged to live with former base hospital nurses in New York. The Andersons, who felt sorry that social stigma forced Grace to leave them so soon, assured her of their help and support.

While at home Grace revealed the details of her months in the army and her parents updated her on the news of all the Andersons. She personally delivered flowers to Clarence's grave and told her brother the "oceans of things," as promised in her letters. As she poured out her heart to Clarence, an avalanche of emotions carried her into the closure she had sought since his death.

Grace left Red Wing hoping to visit again as soon as her personal life improved. She covered thousands of miles from Germany to France, across the Atlantic and then to Minnesota. Tired but tenacious, Grace resolved to be surefooted on the steep trek ahead. She looked forward to a time when society no longer seared brands of shame on women.

In Manhattan her base hospital friends welcomed Grace as their roommate. She cherished the lasting friendships she and the other women had made during the war. The nurses willingly assisted one another because some of them suffered damaged health and postwar depression. Many struggled to resume normal stateside routines after accomplishing their daunting tasks in Europe. Since most family members could not relate to their stressful experiences in the Great War, the nurses confided in and consoled each other.[9]

In Grace's situation, her friends understood the realities of romances where thousands of women worked around hundreds of thousands of men. The nurses, influenced by the conventions of the era and their concern for someone's reputation, never discussed intimate relationships. Grace counted on her friends' discretion while they searched for her nursing position, one with as much anonymity as possible.[9]

Through their base unit contacts at Bellevue Hospital, the nurses found Grace a job in the office of a Bellevue obstetrician. The private office kept her out of public view at the busy hospital.

While Grace cared for obstetrical patients, George handled surgery cases at Camp Hospital No. 33. In late August the AEF relieved George from further duty. The commanding officer of the Pontanezen casual depot put him on the list for departure by "first available government transportation."[10] Because of a delay in transports, George checked the shipping schedule regularly.

September 20, 1919
To: Lieut. Hay, Personnel Section
Casual Depot, Pontanezen
Dear Hay,
    The bearer, Captain George D. Wells, M.C., is the officer I phoned you about. I will regard it as a personal favor if you will register and hold him for the "Orizaba."
    If you will permit him to live in town, I will be personally responsible for his appearing O.K. when called upon to report for this boat.
    L.A.Duff, 1st Lt. C.A.G.
    Orizaba is due the 25th. Load about 26th. Please put him #1 on your list. L.D.[10]

In late September, after a year in Europe, George sailed on the *Orizaba*. On October 15 he reached the port of embarkation headquarters in Hoboken and proceeded to Camp Dix, New Jersey. George requested a short leave of absence before following his orders for an army discharge at Camp Pike in Arkansas.

When George visited Grace they were thankful they both returned safely. Grace's health was excellent and her doctor estimated mid-November as her delivery date. Since George needed to travel to Camp Pike and to his family in Missouri, their relationship remained unsettled. Grace focused on the certainty, the last weeks of her pregnancy, rather than uncertainties.

After his trip to Missouri, George decided to stay in the army. At Camp Pike, a demobilization center, George initially supervised checkups for troops at the medical examining station. On November 3, he reported to the commanding officer of Infirmary No.16, Auxiliary Remount Depot No. 317.

On November 11, the first anniversary of the World War I armistice, Grace gave birth to a baby girl, who she named Martha

Rose. Ever since she contracted Spanish influenza in Germany, she worried about the disease affecting her baby. As soon as the physician pronounced Martha Rose healthy, Grace celebrated a truce in her troubled life.

Grace's friends showered her and Martha Rose with attention and gifts. Grace enjoyed her Thanksgiving and Christmas with Martha Rose and her doting "aunts." She appreciated everything they did for her but she wished George and the Andersons had also shared in the baby's holiday season.

At the start of a new year and a new decade Grace and George made life-changing decisions. In January Grace and her friends parted as she and Martha Rose boarded a westbound train. In 1918 Grace journeyed between Little Rock and New York and voyaged to the Great War. In less than two years she and her two-month-old daughter traveled from New York to Arkansas.

George met Grace and Martha Rose at the Little Rock train station. A few days later they climbed the steps of an impressive 1880s building resembling the medieval architecture in Europe. Inside the Romanesque Revival style structure they kept appointments with the county clerk and the justice of the peace. Grace and George ex-

Grace and George were married January 20, 1920 in the County of Pulaski Courthouse, Arkansas. (57)

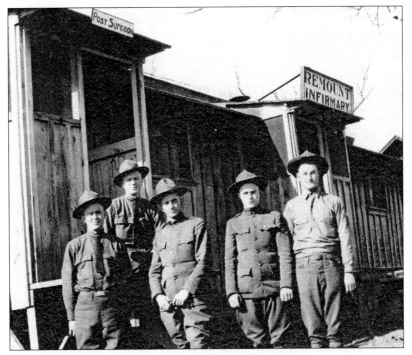

Capt. George Wells, post surgeon, third from left, with other Auxiliary Remount Depot personnel at Camp Pike outside his office and the Remount Infirmary. (58)

changed vows in a quiet civil ceremony at the County of Pulaski courthouse on January 20, 1920.[11]

George and his first wife agreed that a divorce was best for both of them but they were concerned how it would affect Mollie, their five-year-old daughter. Fortunately, Mollie's excitement about having a baby half sister, Martha Rose, eased the tension of both families.

Grace and George began their life together as members of the active military community. George received an honorable discharge from his emergency commission as captain and the appointment as a Medical Corps captain in the regular army. He performed surgery at Camp Pike hospital where, coincidentally, Grace taught nurses anesthesia administration in 1918.

George served as post surgeon of the Auxiliary Remount Depot, one of thirty-nine remount depots the Quartermaster Corps maintained in the postwar period. He managed the sanitary condition of the depot and the health of the men who procured, processed, trained, and issued horses and mules for military use. In the war over a half million horses and mules in the remount system evacuated the wounded and hauled ammunition, water, food, and artillery.[12]

In April Grace, George, and Martha Rose attended the fiftieth wedding anniversary of Fredrick and Ellen Anderson in Red Wing. Grace introduced George and Martha Rose to her father and mother, her siblings, the grandchildren, and other relatives. Grace considered her parents' golden year festivities as a doubly joyful occasion. She returned to Red Wing as a wife and mother less than a year after social stigma ran her out of town.

Back at Camp Pike, additional events of 1920 captured Grace's attention. The lobbying of the Army Nurse Corps eventually produced some results. The Army Reorganization Act of June 4, 1920, recognized the more than twenty thousand World War I army nurses and granted them the status of an officer. Army nurses could wear the insignia of relative rank, from second lieutenant to major, but without the full rights and privileges equal to those of an officer of comparable grade. The ANC pledged to persevere in its appeals.[13]

During the five months leading up to August, Grace and women across the nation watched and waited for the necessary thirty-sixth state to ratify the Nineteenth Amendment. Thirty-five states confirmed from June 1919 through March 1920. In June Delaware unexpectedly defeated the amendment and no other states had legislative sessions scheduled before the November 1920 presidential election.[14]

President Wilson asked the governors of North Carolina and Tennessee to call special sessions. North Carolina defeated the amendment and a spirited debate sparked a political battle in Nashville. The Tennessee senate quickly ratified the amendment. The house, two votes short, fought furiously and the second vote resulted in a tie. A third vote broke the tie. Finally on August 26, 1920, the Nineteenth Amendment became U.S. law.[14]

As a member of the newly formed League of Women Voters, Grace encouraged women to take advantage of their new responsibility. On November 2, 1920, all American women could vote in a presidential election for the first time in history. Republican candidate Warren G. Harding defeated the Democratic opponent, James M. Cox, in an unprecedented landslide win with more than 60 percent of the popular vote.

Grace and George celebrated Martha Rose's first birthday on November 11, the second anniversary of the armistice, and their first Thanksgiving and Christmas as a family. During her Arkansas Christmas in 1917, Grace never dreamed that she would live at Camp Pike three years later with her army officer husband and their daughter.

The next year the War Department ordered George to accompany the Third Division from Camp Pike to Camp Lewis in Tacoma, Washington. Grace and George regretted leaving Arkansas, a state closer to Mollie in Missouri and to the Andersons in Minnesota. However, they served at duty stations on both sides of the Atlantic and thought the Pacific Coast would offer them a new adventure.

At the Camp Lewis cantonment World War I construction crews built a city of over one thousand structures for sixty thousand men. The recruits occupied the barracks on September 5, 1917.[15] Four years later, also in September, the Wells family arrived at Camp Lewis. The Ninth Corps commanding general assigned George to the regimental headquarters at the camp.

The letter Grace wrote on February 11 was the only saved correspondence after her June 1919 telegram to her parents from New York. Grace referred to George by his middle name, Dillard.

Tacoma, Washington - Feb. 11, 1922

Dear Mamma & Papa,

Right after the holidays we moved into camp and I've been so busy trying to settle my quarters. We are very comfortable, have a big living room, a dining room, two big bedrooms, kitchen, bath and a little laundry room with two small stationary tubs, a big front porch and a big back porch. The back porch is big enough to hang my washing out on, ten feet wide and thirty feet long.

Made a very good looking dining room set by painting a home made table and common chairs black. Then painted a little bunch of nasturtiums on the backs of the black chairs, put an old blue rug on the floor and old gold curtains at the windows.

It is awfully pretty really and the whole room cost about forty dollars, rug, curtains & all. It is lots of fun fixing up. Our living room is nice too, really a pretty room and very comfortable. Our bedrooms are not finished.

We have a soldier's wife to help me, she does my washing and helps with the baby. I don't seem to be as husky as I used to be somehow. The baby demands so much of my strength. Guess all women have the same story to tell.

Thank you for the recipes Mamma, and while I think of it I want to ask you for a couple of others, the one for your meatballs fried in deep fat and the one for your veal loaf. Also cracker pudding.

How is the mill coming, Papa? Hope they are not working you too hard. I think of you so often. The weather here seems very mild to me, and is, compared to Minnesota. Dillard thinks it is cold. He is comparing it with southern Missouri, you see.

I love it here. Am very contented. Martha is growing fast and is sweeter all the time. Well I must stop, it is getting late, almost eleven o'clock. It is hard to write letters in the day time. Dearest love to you both from Dillard, Martha, and Grace

As commanding officer of the regimental headquarters detachment, George managed a medical laboratory section, and also ambulance, sanitary, and hospital companies. In 1922 the army added physical examinations, transportation, and regimental supply to his responsibilities.

In August George and nineteen other officers and enlisted men obtained permission to participate in a polo match and horse show in Vancouver, British Columbia. They transported twenty-two "public animals," private mounts, and rations on the August 14-28 trip. The orders said: "The journey is to be accomplished without expense to the government for men or animals."[16]

Following the polo event in Canada, George heard rumors about a reduction in commissioned personnel. A series of events occurred in rapid-fire succession. On September 1 the army relieved George and other Camp Lewis officers of their positions.

Since many World War I veterans were going to California, George and Grace discussed that possibility. In the early 1920s the state beckoned thousands of people with sunshine and a fresh beginning. Some of Grace's relatives including her sister, Joe, and her physician husband, Dr. Wells Howard, moved to the Los Angeles area. They raved about the region.

Five days later George asked for a leave of absence until December 15, 1922, and gave the army a temporary address in Long Beach, California. After his more than five-year career as a U.S. Army Medical Corps officer, George planned to resume his private medical practice. He wrote the State Board of Medical Examiners in Sacramento:

> In the course of a few months I am leaving the military
> service, and it is my desire to practice in the state of Califor-
> nia. I am at present registered in Missouri, and understand
> that state enjoys reciprocal privileges with yours.[17]

On September 14 George received confidential War Department orders announcing his "honorable discharge from the service with one year's pay under the provisions of the Act of Congress approved June 30, 1922, to take effect December 15, 1922." The army instructed George to report to Ross Field, Arcadia, California, on December 15, 1922, "for the accomplishment of your discharge and final settlement of your account."[18]

Tempted by the allure of California, Grace and George set out on a southbound journey of over one thousand miles along the Pacific coast. Their transition back to civilian life and a postwar boom awaited them in Los Angeles.

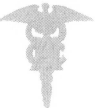

CHAPTER 9

Living as
Civilians in California

*Martha Rose is so lively and wise ... Dr. Wells goes
day and night, and I think has a good future.*[1]
—Grace Anderson Wells

Los Angeles lured newcomers from across the country with its
splendid climate and scenic charms soon after becoming a city and
part of the United States in 1850. Settlers arrived in prairie schoo-
ners, cultivated the rich soil, and harvested abundant crops. Agri-
culture, especially oranges, plus oil discoveries and other opportunities spurred several influxes and land booms. Railroads linked the
continent, promoted Los Angeles, and filled trains with passengers.
Eventually families drove their Ford Model Ts to the fresh Pacific
air and prosperity.

The post-World War I migration more than doubled the Los
Angeles population of nearly 577,000 to over 1.2 million. During
the 1920s most new residents relocated from Midwest farms and
cities. Grace and George Wells, both midwesterners, found their
way to sunny climes in 1922 after five years at army duty stations in
the United States and Europe. The glowing reports that enticed
them to California proved true.

In Long Beach Grace and George visited Signal Hill, covered with tall wooden derricks and wells. A year earlier an oil discovery revealed the largest field ever known in Southern California, already a productive region for "black gold."[2] In Los Angeles they saw the famous orange groves and myriad crops flourishing. Airplanes took off from private landing fields and Hollywood moviemakers filmed the ocean, beaches, mountains, and other natural landscapes.

In December George reported for his army discharge at Ross Field, formerly a World War I army balloon school. During the war, crews learned how to observe simulated artillery fire, make maps, stake out targets, and watch for fighter aircraft.[3] With his approved paperwork in hand, George officially joined the area's burgeoning veteran populace.

From the late 1880s, Los Angeles welcomed veterans with sunshine and an impressive home built by the federal government for disabled Civil War soldiers in Sawtelle, near Santa Monica. Grace and George met the men at the National Soldiers' Home and toured their spacious community, a popular stop for locals and travelers going to the beach.[4]

Gardens, orchards, farmlands, and livestock surrounded elegant Victorian structures – domiciles, infirmaries, staff quarters, mess halls, and a chapel. Private owners, Senator John Percival Jones of Nevada, Col. Robert S. Baker, and his wife, Arcadia DeBaker, deeded the seven hundred acres to the federal government. The donors stipulated that the land, where sheep once grazed, be used in perpetuity for veterans. The soldiers' stories and their Victorian village captivated Grace, who promised to return to Sawtelle often.[4]

Grace and George considered various locales and chose to live southeast of downtown Los Angeles in Bell, part of the thirty-thousand-acre Rancho San Antonio. A land boom between 1870 and 1890 divided the sprawling ranch into smaller holdings. George started his medical practice in Bell in the midst of post-World War I explosive growth when houses and businesses multiplied rapidly.

George opened his office in 1923 and during the next two years the local newspaper printed its first issues and the movie theater screened the new talking motion pictures.[5]

The letters Grace wrote to her parents described Los Angeles in the early 1920s – mostly the same today, from real estate and roses to business problems and backyard fruit trees.

Bell, Calif. - May 8, '23
Dear Mamma & Papa,

Here it is Tuesday morning, ironing day, but everything must wait today till I write you a letter. Trying to get ahead a little, and so we are buying the little house we are in. We can sell it any time we want to, and at least get our rent money back and the small payment we make down.

We are improving it ourselves and they are building new houses all around us which increase the value of this. We just sold two lots that we bought four months ago. We put in less than $150 and got $488 out of it. Pretty good interest don't you think?

The grass and everything burns right up in the sun. I am trying hard to make a lawn and am succeeding fairly well. My flowers grow and bloom fine. I have about sixteen rose bushes started and five of them are blooming already. I started them from twigs I broke off from bushes in January. Geraniums grow like weeds. You don't ever need to water them. Just break off a piece and put it in the ground – and they grow and bloom continually. I am going to send you some to put in the cemetery.

Margaret & Arthur or Fred & Nell [Grace's brothers and their wives] will take you up and put them in for you. I would like to have flowers from my home that I have raised myself on the graves, especially Clarence's. Ella [her cousin] and her family – Auntie [Ella's mother] too, was over here Sunday. We enjoy being in reach of relatives.

Martha Rose was riding her kiddie car last evening & Dillard asked her to let the little boy next door sit on too. But she wouldn't and so her daddy asked her why. She said "Daddy, cause I'm a reckless driver."

All for this time. Oceans of love from Dillard & Martha Rose and Grace

Bell, Calif.- Nov. 18, '23

Dear Mamma and Papa,

Here it is almost Thanksgiving Day again. Washing, ironing, cleaning, sewing – I do it all and there is never enough time. We are well. Still have lots of sunshine and warm weather, too warm in the sun. No rain – lots of dust.

Ella and her family are fine and Joe [her sister] and hers are too. I go to see them nearly every week. Martha Rose has begun to grow fast. Shall send you pictures.

We are just working hard all the time and not going out very much, but feel there is going to be a future here. I am saving and planning to take a trip to see you just as soon as is possible – think I can get rates in the spring. Marian [her niece] tells me you are looking fine and she added "Grandpa is sure frisky." It made me feel awfully good to hear that.

I wish you could live here with me during the cold weather, all the time for that matter. We have an extra bedroom, you would be so welcome. Dillard and I would both love to have you with us. Won't you come? If I take the trip there (which I fully expect to do) then you plan on coming back and spending the winter, or as long as you want.

I know father always wanted his own home. Our lot is big enough for another house too. It could even be arranged to put up a cozy little cottage of your own right here.

Think it over and talk it over, and maybe you will like the idea after awhile. Love to all the "folks" and especially to you, from us all, Grace

Dear Mamma,

Your letter came just as I finished writing this. Was so glad to hear. Joe came over last night and brought me the "State Fair" copy of the Republican, Red Wing Daily. Was much interested to see the pictures of the business men of the town – if the names had not been over the pictures, I would not have known some of them, they have changed so much.

Funny, isn't it, how some people live always in one place and others seem fated to move about so much. I think of no one location any more, in my life, but the world in general. Not from choice, but things have so developed and I have lived in so many places. Of course, I will always be most interested in Red Wing. Much love, Grace

Bell, Calif. - Jan. 14, '24
Dear Mamma and Papa,

Here it is the middle of January already, and my New Year's letters are not yet written. Am glad you had a nice Christmas, wish you could have been with us. It was the happiest Christmas I have had for some time. Not an elaborate Christmas but just cozy and happy and less worries than we have had for some time. Either less worries, or I am learning to trust more in God's goodness. I have prayed my way thru many a hard place and now feel satisfied and confident.

Martha Rose received her card first and she said

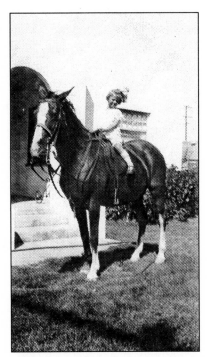

Martha Rose, about three-years-old, posed in the front yard of the Wells home in Los Angeles. She enjoyed riding the horses of "Daddy Doc," her nickname for George. (59)

very confidentially, "Mother, maybe Grandma will send me a box, too. You see she sent me such a nice card." Then when the box came, she said, "My gracious, I'm so surprised! My gracious, I'm so surprised!" all the time she was opening it. She sat right down and strung the beads. She wears them when she dresses up.

She wants a grandma so bad that she plays I am her grandma. Poor little mite. Martha Rose is so lively and wise. I enjoy her so much and love her beyond words. Tell me the ages of Arthur's and Fred's and Floyd's [her brothers] children when you write, will you Mamma? I want to have Martha Rose send them some little gifts some time. I have been away so long I have forgotten how old they would be by now.

Margaret's [sister-in-law] gift was so cute. Martha Rose won't eat with any other knife and fork and feels so important with a case to put them in, that is just like mother's. Nell and Fred [her brother and wife] sent her a beautiful little book.

We are having a cold winter for California. Frost nearly every night. We wish you a Happy New Year, Mamma and Papa, and many more. I am hoping we can get back to see you this year. I am working toward that end. Joe and her family and Dillard and Martha Rose and I were all at Ella's for dinner Sunday night, last.

Good night, now, and much love from Martha Rose, Dillard and Grace

Bell, Calif. - Sept. 25, '24
Dear Mamma & Papa,

I am sending a package of ripe figs home for you to see. They are so delicate, they will perhaps be all smashed when you get them but I thought I would try to send them anyway. I am putting up quince jelly and preserving figs today. It is a big job for me, because I haven't done much of it.

Hope you are well. We are, but working all the time. Dr. Wells goes day and night, and I think has a good future. Wells

Jr. [her nephew] stopped here this morning and said everyone is fine in Long Beach. Must go back to my fruit now. Much love from us all - Martha Rose, Dillard and Grace

Bell, Calif. - Dec. 15, '24
Dear Mamma & Papa,

Don't think I am not thinking of you when I don't write. I think of you every day and want to write but I just put it off. We are so upset. Dr. Wells has had business troubles – got in with the wrong kind of a partner and now is getting away from him, but it is taking all we can rake and scrap together to get rid of him; but it is going to be for the best I am sure. But I am working hard to help.

Christmas can't be much for us this year. Misfortunes have a way of coming right when you want money the most. But anyway I expect to get my trip back to see you by spring. We are all well and so is Joe's family and Ella's. Much love to you all, Grace

Bell, Calif. - Feb. 7, '25
Dear Mamma & Papa,

Well, it is raining here today, and has drizzled most of the week, which is very unusual. Rain is such a treat out here that you never hear anyone say "bad weather" when it rains, but they all say "Isn't this a nice rain."

Martha Rose has been in the house most of the time since Christmas, because she had her tonsils removed right after Xmas, and the poor little thing had so much trouble with her ears. And then after that she caught a cold, so I have fussed with her and nursed her about all the time.

Thank you so much for the lovely Xmas box. Martha Rose says "Thank you, Grandma and Grandpa, for sending me such a nice dolly and everything. The dolly's name is Betty, and I love her very much."

She does, too. She really needed a new doll this year. And

that is just the right kind of a doll for her. Well made and not breakable. She felt very important about sending Grandpa and Grandma the fruit cake, and told everybody. She wants to see you so bad. I suppose because I have talked to her so much.

We are hoping and trusting that we can come home to see you this next summer. If business only opens up better and we think it surely will. Guess we have a lot to be thankful for, that we can keep going. Lots of people have gone broke – had to go out of business this year.

Hope you are still well and happy. All our love to you and many kisses from Martha Rose, Grace

Bell, Calif. - May 18, '25
Dear Mamma and Papa,

Mother's Day, but I shall include you both in this letter. I meant to have a letter reach you for today, but it crept up on me before I realized it and I woke up to find today is Mother's Day. I hope you are having a Happy Day and wish I were with you.

Martha Rose and I are still planning on getting home this summer, and expect to leave here the first of July. I am sewing and working hard to that end.

We are all well, so is Joe's family and Ella's. All our love to dear Mother and Father - Dillard, Martha Rose and Grace

Bell, Calif. - Nov. 7, '25
Dear Mamma and Papa,

I have been home for about two weeks and have been sick, so has Martha Rose. We caught cold in Kansas City. Dr. Wells had ordered the painters to come and paint the house and I've had to work right with them and watch to see it was done right.

Mother dear, I am sending you a lace collar for your birthday that I think is just the shape you want. This letter is only to let you know we got through all right and wish you many happy returns of your birthday. Will write more news soon as I get these painters off my hands. Write when you can. Much love from us all, Martha Rose & Grace

Grace continued traveling to Minnesota to see her parents who remained in Red Wing and never wintered in Los Angeles. In 1932 her father passed on at age eighty-seven and in 1936 her mother died at age eighty-eight.

The *Red Wing Republican Daily* gave Fredrick this tribute: "One of the county's highly respected and hardy pioneers, who helped to lay the foundations of a prosperous and happy community ... a citizen of sterling character, who was respected by all who knew him."[6] The newspaper lauded Ellen as "one of the city's beloved pioneer women ... a kindly and charitable woman, whose chief interests in life were her church and her home... her passing will bring sorrow to many."[7]

Grace's prediction that George "has a good future" became a reality. Business improved, as they believed it would. George's medical practice expanded beyond Bell to neighboring Vernon, where he established the Wells Industrial Emergency Hospital. The Wells facility served the exclusively industrial city's large labor force from companies including Farmer John, Swift, U.S. Steel, Bethlehem Steel, Alcoa, Owens-Illinois Glass, and American Can.[8]

George, a member of the surgical staff at Los Angeles County Hospital, held offices in the Los Angeles County Medical Association and the local branch of the American Medical Association. His membership in the Los Angeles Athletic Club and the Los Angeles Chamber of Commerce drew a variety of patients to his practice, from downtown business executives to athletes, especially fellow polo players. George's Quartermaster Corps remount depot duty led to owning polo horses and playing the sport for recreation.

Their early 1920s lifestyle of "just working hard all the time and not going out very much" changed dramatically for Grace and George. They attended shows featuring the award-winning art of

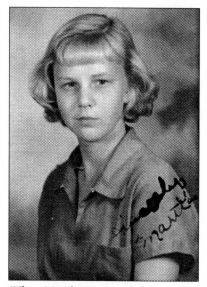

When Martha Rose signed her school photo in bottom right corner, she smudged the word sincerely. (60)

Joe, Grace's sister, whose paintings were displayed in prominent California and U.S. galleries. George's affiliation with medical associations, the Shriners, Elks, and Veterans of Foreign Wars involved them in social, cultural, and philanthropic activities.

Grace and George liked living a short drive from major events at the Los Angeles Memorial Coliseum, which was being built when they arrived and opened in 1923. They enjoyed the 1932 Summer Olympics (Xth Olympiad) and the annual Armistice Day commemoration with throngs of spectators, thousands of World War I veterans marching in a parade, taps at 11 a.m., a band concert, and other ceremonies.[9] The Wells family regarded Armistice Day, also Martha Rose's birthday, as a significant personal occasion as well as a patriotic one.

Since Grace's devotion to wounded soldiers never wavered, she kept her promise to the veterans at Sawtelle. She went to the National Soldiers' Home to listen to their war stories and tell them a few of her own. During the 1920s the facility enlarged to meet the needs of World War I veterans and the Victorian community closed. In the 1930s and afterwards Grace visited veterans on the original federal property at the modern VA Wadsworth Center, also a teaching hospital for the UCLA Medical School.[10]

Their first small house and two lots Grace and George bought and sold in Bell snowballed into various real estate holdings. Eventually they purchased a Spanish-style ranch home, surrounded by enough acreage for polo horses and extra land they gradually sold as residential lots.

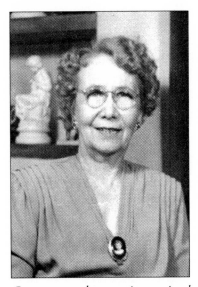

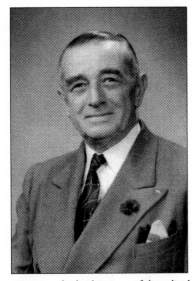

Grace returned to nursing, assisted George at their hospital, and continued visiting the veterans at VA Wadsworth Center. (61)

George, who built a successful medical practice, was active in medical associations, the Shriners, Elks, and Veterans of Foreign Wars. (62)

At their rancho they entertained local relatives and friends as well as out-of-towners such as former Base Hospital No. 115 nurses. Family members living nearby increased as Grace's brother, George's three sisters, and others moved west. Martha Rose and Mollie, George's older daughter and their favorite and most frequent guest, formed a close friendship. While the half sisters were growing up and into adulthood, they exchanged letters and spent summer vacations together in Missouri and California.

When Martha Rose entered college to major in business, Grace obtained her California certification as a registered nurse. When Grace met George at the Vichy Hospital Center, she never imagined that some day they would treat patients at their own emergency hospital. They even trained Martha Rose to assist with bookkeeping, medical dictation, and minor surgery.

During World War II Grace and George demonstrated their patriotism once again. They took part in civil defense drills and recycled metal, paper, and rubber. They invested in war bonds and

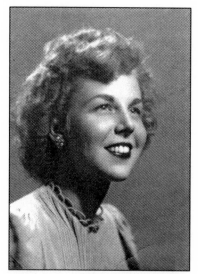

Martha Rose, a business major in college, helped with bookkeeping and medical dictation at the Wells Emergency Hospital. (63)

used ration cards for gasoline, meat, coffee, and sugar. Martha Rose, one of the hundreds of thousands of women in the home front workforce, utilized her college business skills as an executive secretary at Alcoa's Los Angeles reduction plant. George volunteered as an examining physician in the U.S. Selective Service System.

Twenty-seven years after Grace encountered "the wildest thing imaginable" in Vichy on Armistice Day, she participated in the revelry on V-J Day in 1945. Bedlam broke out throughout Los Angeles as sirens, auto horns, and boat whistles blared. Paper scraps rained down from office building windows as crowds rushed into the streets to dance, parade, and cheer the victory all day and night. Following World War II, to the delight of Grace and the Army Nurse Corps, the nurses became eligible for all the GI Bill veteran benefits.[11]

Two Wells family celebrations also occurred in 1945. Grace and George marked their twenty-fifth wedding anniversary. Martha Rose married Charles Swan, a U.S. Navy Reserve veteran, the son of Dr. Alfred H. Swan, a Southern California surgeon.

Exciting national news caught Grace's attention in 1947. Finally, after serving in two world wars, the Army Nurse Corps received the full benefits and privileges of their rank. The Army-Navy Nurse Act of 1947 provided ANC members with permanent commissioned officer status in the grades of second lieutenant through lieutenant colonel. Congress also established the Army Nurse Corps in the Medical Department of the regular army.[11]

A postwar population explosion brought thousands of veterans to Los Angeles, where they were stationed or passed through during World War II. The boom produced more patients for George's practice and the Wells hospital. George stepped up his pace but his hectic schedule took its toll.

On February 9, 1948, George suffered a heart attack. Grace stayed by her husband's side as the doctors tried desperately using every treatment available at the time to save their colleague. Sadly, George spent only twelve hours in the hospital and died of cardiac failure two months before his sixty-third birthday.

Although losing the love of her life shocked and devastated Grace, she felt grateful for their nearly thirty-year marriage and for being beside George in his last hours. Grace planned two services, one in Los Angeles and another in Missouri, for the interment. Observing a Wells family tradition, she buried her husband at Shiloh Cemetery near Springfield, close to the graves of his parents and siblings.

When companies sent letters to Grace expressing condolences and gratitude for the emergency hospital, she decided to keep the facility functioning. Martha Rose helped with bookkeeping and

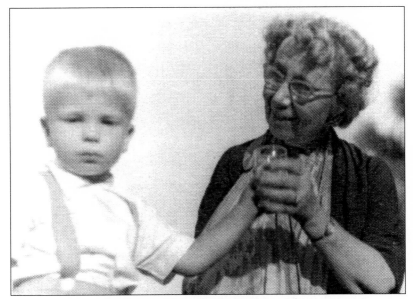

Grace retired to spend more time with
her grandson, Dana, three-years-old, in 1953. (64)

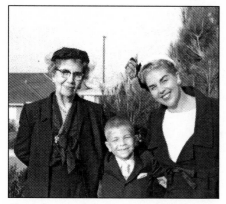

Grace, her grandson, Dana, and Martha Rose, enjoyed a special occasion in the 1950s.(65)

additional duties for two years, until the birth of her son, Dana, in 1950. A few years later Grace sold the hospital and retired so she could spend more time with her daughter and grandson.

Grace volunteered at the VA Wadsworth Hospital and with the League of Women Voters for local and national elections. She followed important Army Nurse Corps news including the ANC working in MASH units in the Korean War and both male and female ANC members serving in the Vietnam War.[12] Grace never tired of new adventures like flying rather than taking the train. She flew to New York and elsewhere for her base hospital reunions, to Red Wing to see relatives, to George's gravesite in Missouri, and U.S. and Canadian locales for vacations.

Martha Rose, active as a PTA parent, a church schoolteacher, and charity drive worker while Dana was in school, pursued her business career again after her divorce. She served as her mother's caregiver for five years until 1973, the year Grace passed away at age eighty-eight.

Grace's memorial marker at the Veteran Affairs Los Angeles National Cemetery reflects the military rank the Army Nurse Corps sought and finally received. Her niche plaque reads: Grace M. Wells, Minn., Lt. Nurse Corps Army, WWI. Grace and over 84,000 other veterans are interred at the 114-acre cemetery, dedicated in 1889 and located on the same property as the former National Soldiers' Home.[13]

At "The Arlington of the West" numerous rows of white headstones stand like a massive army on expansive lawns. Streets named for battlefields such as Gettysburg, Antietam, Belleau Wood, and Argonne lead to graves, monuments, a rose garden, and the Bob

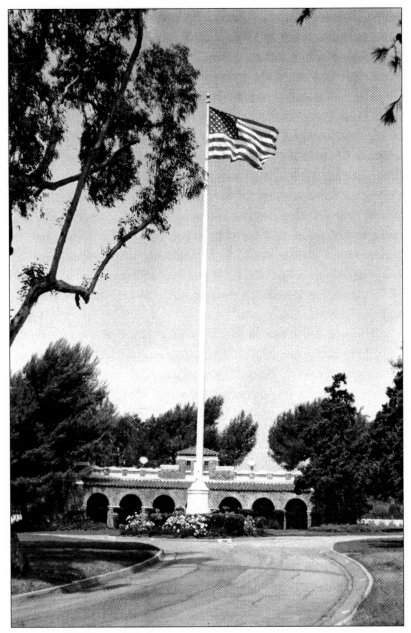

*An American flag flies high over the indoor columbarium of the
Veteran Affairs Los Angeles National Cemetery. Grace's niche plaque reads:
Grace M. Wells, Minn., Lt. Nurse Corps Army, WWI. (66)*

Hope Veterans Chapel. Chateau Thierry Avenue and Marne Avenue curve together at Grace's final resting place in the Spanish revival-style indoor columbarium. Nearby an American flag, visible from every section of the graveyard, flies atop a towering pole.

The nineteenth century cemetery and the VA Greater Los Angeles Healthcare System, with dozens of buildings spread across nearly four hundred acres, occupy most of the seven hundred acres gifted to the federal government in 1887 for the benefit of veterans. The Veterans Park Conservancy, which protects the irreplaceable open space from commercial development, completed the first phase of a sixteen-acre Los Angeles National Veterans Park in 2006. The oasis, in the midst of a crowded urban area, will combine natural beauty and a history walk. As envisioned, people of all ages will celebrate America and the achievements and sacrifices of veterans while they enjoy flowering meadows, butterfly gardens, grassy knolls, and century-old eucalyptus.[13]

If Grace Anderson Wells were alive today, she undoubtedly would praise the patriotic spirit and efforts of the people who are creating the national place of honor. The veterans park evokes the same devotion to servicemen and women in the twenty-first century as the stirring lyrics of the unit song, "Pride of America, We're With You," sung in 1918 by Grace and the World War I nurses of Base Hospital No. 115.

End Notes

Introduction

1. "When we get ready to sail ...": Grace Matilda Anderson, "Grace Anderson Letters, 1917-1925," July 22, 1918, Anderson Wells Memorabilia, private collection.

2. "We nurses are provided ...": Ibid., August 1918.

3. "We'll soon be with you ...": "Unit No. 115 Song," Ibid., July 22, 1918.

4. Army nurses in Europe: Mary T. Sarnecky, Col. USA (Ret.), *A History of the U.S. Army Nurse Corps* (Philadelphia: University of Pennsylvania Press, 1999), 122 (10,245 Army Nurse Corps nurses in France); Col. Joseph H. Ford, M.C., *The Medical Department of the United States Army in the World War*, vol. 2, *Administration American Expeditionary Forces* (Washington, DC: GPO, 1927), chap. 7, 127, (10,081 nurses served in the American Expeditionary Forces), available online at http://history.amedd.army.mil/booksdocs/wwi/adminamerexp/default.htm.

5. "I would be very happy here ...": "Anderson Letters," December 6, 1918.

6. "a kick or a knock": Ibid., December 6, 1918.

7. "a real breakfast ...": Ibid., November 12, 1918.

8. "packed in like sardines ...": Ibid., November 12, 1918.

9. "people shouting ...": Ibid., November 14, 1918.

10. "Germans stop ...": Ibid., February 14, 1919.

11. "We started from Fredrickshald ...": Andreas Fredrick Andersen, "Biography of the Andersens," 1927, 1, Anderson Wells Memorabilia.

12. "out against the Indians . . . ": Ibid, 2.

13. Early years of Ellen Anderson: Ellen Anderson obituary, *Red Wing (MN) Republican Daily,* April 9, 1936; Andersen, "Biography," 2.

14. Fredrick Andersen: Andersen, "Biography," 1-2.

15. Survivor of *Sea Wing*: Arthur Anderson obituary, *Red Wing (MN) Republican Eagle Daily*, August 5, 1959.

16. *Sea Wing* Disaster: Minnesota Historical Society, "Sea Wing Disaster," http://www.mnhs.org/school/online/communities/milestones/milestones_sea_wing_disaster.htm.

17. "Pride of America ...": Unit No. 115 song, "Anderson Letters," July 22, 1918.

Chapter One

1. "I am very glad . . . ready for anything.": "Anderson Letters," July 10, 1918.

2. U.S. assistance, neutrality: Lettie Gavin, *American Women in World War I: They Also Served* (Niwot: University Press of Colorado, 1997), 44-45; Dorothy and Carl J. Schneider, *Into the Breach: American Women Overseas in World War I* (New York: Viking Penguin, 1991), 4, 81-82, 87; Brig. Peter Young, ed. in chief, *The Marshall Cavendish Illustrated Encyclopedia of World War I,* 12 vols. (New York: Marshall Cavendish, 1984), 11:3418.

3. U.S. entry into war: Simon Adams, *Eyewitness Books: World War I* (New York: Dorling Kindersley, 2001), 54; Woodrow Wilson, "War Message to Congress," April 2, 1917, Brigham Young University Library, http://www.lib.byu.edu/~rdh/wwi/1917/wilswarm.html.

4. Selective Service: *The Grolier Library of World War I*, 8 vols. (Danbury, CT: Grolier Educational, 1997), 5:56; United States National Archives and Records Administration, "World War I Selective Service System Draft Registration Cards," National Archives and Records Administration, http://www.archives.gov/genealogy/military/ww1/draft-registration/.

5. Committee on Public Information campaign: George Creel, *How We Advertised America* (New York: Harper & Brothers, 1920), 3-9; Museum of Ventura County, Patriotism and Persuasion: Posters of World War I, Ventura, CA, June 3 - August 28, 2005; *Grolier Library*, 5:58-59; Young, *Cavendish Encyclopedia*, 9:2903; Anne Cipriano Venzon, ed., *The United States in the First World War, An Encyclopedia* (New York: Garland Publishing, 1995), 162-64.

6. Selective Service Draft: Venzon, *United States*, 147, 540-42; National Archives, "Selective Service"; Ancestry.com "World War I Draft Registration Cards, 1917-1918," Ancestry.com, http://content.ancestry.com/iexec/?htx=List&dbid=6482&offerid=0:7858:0; United States Department of Defense, "DOD Principal Wars in Which the United States Participated - U.S. Military Personnel Serving and Casualties," http://siadapp.dmdc.osd.mil/personnel/CASUALTY/WCPRINCIPAL.pdf; Doughboy Center, *The Story of the American Expeditionary Forces*, Walter Kudlick, "Sealift Transporting the AEF to Europe," The Great War Society, http://www.worldwar1.com/dbc; Museum of Ventura County, Patriotism; *Grolier Library*, 5:59, 61; C. A. Rasmussen, *History of Red Wing* (Red Wing, MN: privately published, 1933), 178.

7. "100% Americanism," Liberty Bonds, War Savings Stamps, food conservation: Museum of Ventura County, Patriotism; *Grolier Library*, 5:30, 64-65; Young, *Cavendish Encyclopedia*, 9:2904; Venzon, *United States*, 341-42, 776-77; Nancy Gentile Ford, *Americans All! Foreign-born Soldiers in World War I*, (College Station: Texas A&M University Press, 2001), 3, 11, 147; Rasmussen, *History of Red Wing*, 179-80.

8. Anti-German sentiment: Museum of Ventura County, Patriotism; *Grolier Library*, 5:30.

9. Red Cross growth: American Red Cross Museum, "American Red Cross Nursing," "World War I Accomplishments of the American Red Cross," American Red Cross, http://www.redcross.org/museum/history/; Museum of Ventura County, Patriotism.

10. Red Cross recruitment: American Red Cross Museum, "World War I"; Museum of Ventura County, Patriotism.

11. U.S. Army Nurse Corps data: Lt. Col. Carolyn M. Feller, AN, USAR, and Maj. Debora R. Cox, AN, eds., *Highlights in the History of the Army Nurse Corps* (Washington, DC: U.S. Army Center of Military History, 2001), 1901, 1917, 1918; available online at http://www.army.mil/cmh/books/anc-highlights/highlights.htm.

12. Women's suffrage and New Woman: Schneider and Schneider, *Into the Breach*, 1, 4-5; *Grolier Library*, 5:10-11; Young, *Cavendish Encyclopedia*, 11:3418-20; Venzon, *United States*, 803; The Ohio State University Department of History, "Clash of Cultures in the 1910s and 1920s – The New Woman," The Ohio State University Department of History, http://history.osu.edu/projects/Clash/New Woman/newwomen-page1.htm (accessed May 4, 2006; site now discontinued), See http://history.osu.edu/.

13. "I am very glad to go ...": "Anderson Letters," July 10, 1918.

14. General John J. Pershing's cabled request: Feller and Cox, *Highlights*, October 2, 1917; Ford, *Medical Department*, vol. 2, *Administration*, chap. 7, 125.

15. United States Army Nurse Corps Records of Grace M. Anderson, War Department, Office of the Surgeon General, Washington DC, 1917-1919, November 27, 1917, Anderson Wells Memorabilia.

Chapter Two

1. "There are a fine lot of men here ...": "Anderson Letters," January 26, 1918.

2. "No one seems to know ...": Ibid., December 4, 1917.

3. "The road outside . . . ": Ibid., December 10, 1917.

4. Camp Pike, cantonments: Old State House Museum, "Arkansas Camp Has Major Role in the Great War," Old State House Museum, search for Camp Pike at http://www.oldstatehouse.com/; Learning Centers at Ancestry.com, "Chart of World War I National Army Cantonments," Rootsweb.com, http://freepages .military.rootsweb.com/~worldwarone/WWI/Maps/chart.html; Venzon, *United States*, 127; Stanhope Bayne-Jones, MD, *The Evolution of Preventive Medicine in the United States Army, 1607-1939* (Washington, DC: GPO, 1968), 152, available online at http://history.amedd.army.mil/booksdocs/misc/evprev/.

5. Nurses' service, patients at camp hospitals: Sarnecky, *History Army Nurse Corps*, 82; Bayne-Jones, *Evolution Preventive Medicine*, 152.

6. Diversity of World War I troops: Doughboy Center, "Amazing Facts and Remarkable Trivia About the AEF"; *Grolier Library*, 7:82-83; Venzon, *United States*, 87-89, 540; Ford, *Americans All*, 3, 13, 15, 67, 88-90, 108-9; Jami L. Bryan, "Fighting for Respect: African-American Soldiers in WWI," Army History Research, Army Historical Foundation, http:www.armyhistory.org/ armyhistorical.aspx?pgID=868&id=103&exCompID=32.

7. Organizations at camps: Venzon, *United States*, 159-60; Ford, *Americans All*, 9, 96-98, 105.

8. Mayo Clinic observation, army anesthesia training: Virginia S. Thatcher, *History of Anesthesia with Emphasis on the Nurse Specialist* (Philadelphia: J.B. Lippincott, 1953), 56-58, 93-97; Sarnecky, *History Army Nurse Corps*, 129-31; American Association of Nurse Anesthetists, "AANA Overview," "History of Nurse Anesthesia Practice," American Association of Nurse Anesthetists, http://www .aana.com/aboutaana.aspx.

9. Armed Forces insurance: Venzon, *United States*, 776.

10. Maj. Gen. Samuel Sturgis: Arlington National Cemetery, "Samuel Davis Sturgis, Jr.," Arlington National Cemetery, http://www.arlingtoncemetery.net/sturgisj .htm.

11. Trench training: Old State House, "Arkansas Camp."

12. Nurses needed in U.S., Europe: Ford, *Medical Department,* vol. 2, *Administration,* chap. 7, 126; Bayne-Jones, *Evolution Preventive Medicine,* 152.

13. Commission on Training Camp Activities: Venzon, *United States,* 160; Ford, *Americans All,* 97-99.

14. Nurses in Europe and U.S.: Ford, *Medical Department,* vol. 2, *Administration,* chap. 7. 126

15. Army orders: Anderson Army Records, July 9, 1918.

Chapter Three

1. "We drill every day …": "Anderson Letters," July 16, 1918.

2. Troop departure statistics: Doughboy Center, "AEF Fact Sheet," and "Sealift Transporting"; James H. Hallas, ed., *Doughboy War: The American Expeditionary Force in World War I* (Boulder, CO: Lynne Rienner Publishers, 2000), 31; Venzon, *United States,* 749.

3. Slacker raids, *Hearts of the World* and theaters: Venzon, *United States,* 224, 556; *Grolier Library,* 5:61.

4. Nurses' expenses: Sarnecky, *History Army Nurse Corps,* 84.

5. Relative rank: Schneider and Schneider, *Into the Breach,* 109; Venzon, *United States,* 716, 803; Gavin, *American Women,* 43.

6. Base hospitals' totals for patients, beds: Ford, *Medical Department,* vol. 2, *Administration,* chap. 24, 629-748, chap. 16, 312, 314. (A total of 929,740 medical and surgical patients was reported in the patient counts of 108 base hospital histories. When the patients of the other twenty-two base hospitals plus camp hospitals and convalescent camps are added, the total is over 1.3 million.).

7. Base hospital system genesis, Dr. George W. Crile: Sarnecky, *History Army Nurse Corps,* 80-81; Gavin, *American Women,* 44-46. Alexander Bunts and George Crile, Jr., "The Founders," The Cleveland Clinic, http://www.clevelandclinic .org/act/Section1.pdf; John S. O'Shea, MD, "Responding to Crisis: Franklin H. Martin, the ACS, and the Great War," *Bulletin of the American College of Surgeons,* vol. 89, no. 6, The American College of Surgeons, http://www.facs.org/ fellows_info/bulletin/2004/oshea0604.pdf; Bayne-Jones, *Evolution Preventive Medicine,* 151.

8. Base hospital organization: Ford, *Medical Department,* vol. 2, *Administration,* chap. 24, 629-748.

9. U-boats, convoy system: Capt. Dudley W. Knox, "American Naval Participation in the Great War (With Special Reference to the European Theater of Operations)," (Washington DC: Department of the Navy, Naval Historical Center, 2003), parts 1, 2, http://www.history.navy.mil/library/special/american _naval_ part_great_war.htm; *Grolier Library,* vol. 5:50-51; Venzon, *United States,* 43-45.

10. U.S. Navy in World War I: Knox, "American Naval," parts 1-7; Venzon, *United States,* 751.

11. Troop, base hospital transport, shipping capacity: Knox, "American Naval," part 3; Doughboy Center, "Sealift Transporting"; Ford, *Medical Department,* vol. 2, *Administration,* chap. 24, 629-748.

12. Base hospital unit accidents: Ford, *Medical Department*, vol. 2, *Administration*, chap. 24, 635-36, 639-40; Sarnecky, *History Army Nurse Corps*, 82.

13. 1906 voyage: Ellen Matilda Anderson, "Letters from Europe," June 11, 1906, Anderson Wells Memorabilia.

14. Shipboard activities: Sarnecky, *History Army Nurse Corps*, 83; Doughboy Center, "Sealift Transporting."

15. King George V letter: Anderson Wells Memorabilia.

16. U.S. submarines: Knox, *"American Naval,"* part 4; Venzon, *United States,* 750.

17. AEF nurses: Ford, *Medical Department*, vol. 2, *Administration,* chap. 7, 126.

18. Changes for base hospitals, Ibid., chap. 14, 235.

19. Army orders: Anderson Army Records, August 18, 1918.

20. "share your joys …": "Anderson Letter," July 22, 1918

21. "take our chance …": Ibid.

Chapter Four

1. "Our boys are the finest …": "Anderson Letters," October 4, 1918.

2. Second Battle of the Marne: Doughboy Center, "Second Battle of the Marne."

3. Base No. 17 and base hospitals' procurement, location, construction: Ford, *Medical Department*, vol. 2, *Administration*, chap. 14, 233; chap. 15, 271, 280; chap. 24, 636-712.

4. Army Corps of Engineers: Venzon, *United States*, 697-700; Doughboy Center, "Advance Section Services of Supply."

5. U.S. Air Service: Venzon, *United States,* 6-7; Doughboy Center, "American Air Service in the Great War," "AEF Fact Sheet."

6. Second Battle of the Marne: Doughboy Center, "Second Battle of the Marne."

7. Meuse-Argonne Offensive: Doughboy Center, "The Big Show, the Meuse-Argonne Offensive"; Venzon, *United States,* 616.

8. Base Hospital crisis expansion: Ford, *Medical Department*, vol. 2, *Administration*, chap. 16, 288; Gavin, *American Women,* 53.

9. World War I injuries: Hallas, *Doughboy War*, 124, 152, 158; Gavin, *American Women,* 43, 47; *Grolier Library*, 7:30, 53, 76.

10. World War I casualties: Department of Defense, "DOD Principal Wars"; Bayne-Jones, *Evolution Preventive Medicine*, 151.

11. Care of wounded, multiple injuries: Sarnecky, *History Army Nurse Corps,* 96-97; Hallas, *Doughboy War,* 158; Gavin, *American Women,* 43-44, 71-72; Col. Joseph H. Ford, M.C., et al. *The Medical Department of the United States Army in the World War,* vol. 8, *Field Operations* (Washington, DC: GPO, 1925), chap. 5, 159, available online at http://history.amedd.army.mil/booksdocs/wwi/fieldoperations/default.htm.

12. Medical handling procedure: Doughboy Center, "AEF Casualty Handling Procedures"; Hallas, *Doughboy War,* 151-52; Venzon, *United States,* 714; Gavin, *American Women,* 49.

13. Spanish influenza: Hallas, *Doughboy War,* 293-94; Sarnecky, *History Army Nurse Corps,* 120; Jeffery K. Taubenberger and David M. Morens, "1918 Influenza: the Mother of All Pandemics," Centers for Disease Control and Prevention, http:// www.cdc.gov/ncidod/EID/vol12no01/05-0979.htm; Venzon, *United States,* 573-74; Young, *Cavendish Encyclopedia,* 10:2974-75; Gavin, *American Women,* 63; Department of Defense, "DOD Principal Wars"; Bayne-Jones, *Evolution Preventive Medicine,* 152.

14. Services of Supply trains: Doughboy Center, "Amazing Facts." Venzon, *United States,* 697.

15. Army orders: Anderson Army Records, October 3, October 25, 1918.

Chapter Five

1. "It will be quite a long time ...": "Anderson Letters," November 14, 1918.

2. Vichy base hospital center: Ford, *Medical Department,* vol. 2, *Administration,* chap. 16, 286; chap. 21, 476.

3. Base Hospitals at Vichy: Ibid., chap. 24, 629, 646, 695, 728, 732-33.

4. World War I hospital trains: Ibid., chap. 17, 319, 324; chap. 18, 363.

5. Nurses' insufficient number and distribution: Ibid., chap. 21, 482-483.

6. American nurse anesthetists: Sarnecky, *History Army Nurse Corps,* 130; AANA, "History Nurse Anesthesia."

7. Army nurses training at Mayo Clinic: Thatcher, *History of Anesthesia,* 97-98; Sarnecky, *History Army Nurse Corps,* 130-31.

8. Surgeon General, departments of anesthesia: Thatcher, *History of Anesthesia,* 98.

9. Nitrous oxide-oxygen anesthesia: Ibid., 97.

10. Roentgenology Department, Ford, *Medical Department,* vol. 2, *Administration,* chap. 18, 366-67.

11. Reactions to Armistice news: *Grolier Library,* 7:113-117; Adams, *Eyewitness Books,* 60.

12. Deaths of nurses: Feller and Cox, *Highlights,* November 11, 1918; Sarnecky, *History Army Nurse Corps,* 121.

13. Maxillofacial, Neurology, Ophthalmology: Ford, *Medical Department,* vol. 2, *Administration,* chap. 18, 363-64, 367-68, 374-75; chap. 21, 479-80; chap. 27, 810.

14. Army Medical Museum: *The Caduceus,* January 29, 1919, Anderson Wells Memorabilia.

15. Medical consultants: Ford, *Medical Department,* vol. 2, *Administration,* chap.18, 376, 385.

16. Base hospitals arrive: Ibid., chap. 24 (thirty-eight base hospital histories).

17. Inadequate number of base hospitals: Ibid., chap. 16, 286.

18. Nurses awaiting transportation, arrival in France: Ibid., chap. 7, 126-27.

19. Largest number of ANC nurses: Sarnecky, *History Army Nurse Corps,* 122. (10,245 Army Nurse Corps nurses served in France); Ford, *Medical Department,* vol. 2, *Administration,* chap. 7, 127 (10,081- greatest number of nurses in AEF).

20. Base hospital recreation: Ford, *Medical Department*, vol. 2, *Administration*, chap. 21, 487-88.

21. Officers' club: Ibid., list of figures, 122.

22. Social news: *The Caduceus*, January 29, 1919.

23. Vichy Center Christmas Program, Commanding Officer letter: Anderson Wells Memorabilia.

Chapter Six

1. "It is hard to be over here …": "Anderson Letters," January 14 and January 15, 1919.

2. Demobilization, debarkation camps: Venzon, *United States*, 198; *Grolier Library*, 8:20-24; Doughboy Center, "Sealift Transporting."

3. Clarence Anderson: Clarence Anderson Obituary: *Red Wing (MN) Daily Republican*, December 28, 1918.

4. Medical Department demobilization: Ford, *Medical Department*, vol. 2, *Administration*, chap. 14, 236; chap. 27, 807-12.

5. Closure of Base Hospitals: Ibid., chap. 24, 629-748.

6. Vichy Commanding Officer quote: *The Caduceus*, January 29, 1919.

7. American women's morality: Schneider and Schneider, *Into the Breach*, 265.

8. Army orders: Anderson Army Records, February 6, 1919.

9. Army orders: United States Army Medical Corps Records of George Dillard Wells, War Department, Office of the Surgeon General, Washington, DC, 1917 – 1922, February 12, 1919, Anderson Wells Memorabilia.

Chapter Seven

1. "If our boys need us. . .": "Anderson Letters," February 6, 1919.

2. Chateau-Thierry Battle: Doughboy Center, "Chateau-Thierry Overview," "Chateau-Thierry, the Battle for Belleau Wood."

3. Chateau-Thierry battlefield and cemeteries: FirstWorldWar.com, "Touring the Battlefields," "The First Battlefield Tours," FirstWorldWar.com, http://www .firstworldwar.com/tours/firsttours.htm; Chateau-Thierry photos, Anderson Wells Memorabilia.

4. American Third Army: Ford, *Medical Department*, vol. 2, *Administration*, chap. 28, 813; Ford, et al, *Medical Department*, vol. 8, *Field Operations*, chap. 38, 907.

5. Military Police permit: Anderson Wells Memorabilia.

6. Evacuation Hospital No. 26: Ford, *Medical Department*, vol. 2, *Administration*, chap. 28, 815-16; Ford, et al., *Medical Department*, vol. 8, *Field Operations*, chap. 38, 905-6, 908-9.

7. Coblenz Hospital Center: Ibid., vol. 2, *Administration*, chap. 28, 815-16.

8. Germans' welcome: Young, *Cavendish Encyclopedia*, 11:3381, 3383.

9. The Rainbow Division: United States Army Center of Military History, "42nd Infantry Division History," Center of Military History, http://www.42id.army .mil/history/index.html.

10. Mesves Hospital Center: Ford, *Medical Department*, vol. 2, *Administration*, chap. 21, 476.

11. Post-war Germany history: *Grolier Library*, 7:106-7; 8:12, 19; Venzon, *United States*, 33.

12. Base Hospital No. 109, Vichy Hospital Center: Ford, *Medical Department*, vol. 2, *Administration*, chap. 24, 728; chap. 21, 477.

13. Base units' closures, return: Ibid, chap. 24, 629-748.

14. Unwed pregnancy, abortion, single parenting, adoption, divorce: Wilma Mankiller et al, eds., *The Reader's Companion to U.S. Women's History* (New York: Houghton Mifflin, 1998), 4, 269-70; 360-61; 540-42.

15. Army Nurse Corps misconduct: Sarnecky, *History Army Nurse Corps*, 116.

16. Ambulance Companies, Company No. 155, Seventh Corps: Ford et al., *Medical Department*, vol. 8, *Field Operations*, chap. 38, 911, 934-35. Ford, *Medical Department*, vol. 2, *Administration*, chap. 17, 336; chap. 21, 485.

17. Spanish influenza: Taubenberger and Morens, "1918 Influenza"; Venzon, *United States*, 573-74; Young, *Cavendish Encyclopedia*, 9:2974.

18. Ambulance Companies in Germany: Ford, *Medical Department*, vol. 2, *Administration*, chap. 21, 485; Ford et al, *Medical Department*, vol. 8, *Field Operations*, chap. 5, 211.

19. General John J. Pershing to AEF women: Anderson Wells Memorabilia.

20. Hospital closures in Germany: Ford, *Medical Department*, vol. 2, *Administration*, chap 28, 816; Ford, et al, *Medical Department*, vol. 8, *Field Operations*, chap. 38, 908.

21. George D. Wells memos to Chief Surgeon and Commanding General: Wells Army Records, May 11, May 12, 1919.

22. Army Orders: Anderson Army Records, May 9, May 30, 1919.

Chapter Eight

1. "Please wire me ... be home soon.": "Anderson Letters," June 21, 1919.

2. American troops return: Doughboy Center, Kudlick, "Sealift Transporting."

3. Troops post card: Anderson Wells Memorabilia.

4. Army Nurse Corps pay: Anderson Army Records, June 19, 1919.

5. Nineteenth Amendment Passage: Judy Monroe, *The Nineteenth Amendment, Women's Right to Vote* (Springfield, NJ: Enslow Publishers, 1998), 1, 69-72, 74; Marjorie Spruill Wheeler, ed., *One Woman, One Vote: Rediscovering the Woman Suffrage Movement* (Troutdale, OR: NewSage Press, 1995), 333.

6. Relative rank: Schneider and Schneider, *Into the Breach*, 109; Venzon, *United States*, 716.

7. Camp Hospital No. 33: Ford, *Medical Department*, vol. 2, *Administration*, chap. 25, 762-63.

8. Relief from active duty: Anderson Army Records, June 20, August 10, 1919.

9. Nurses' attitudes, post-war problems: Schneider and Schneider, *Into the Breach*, 264, 267, 273-74, 276-77, 281.

10. Relief from duty, Pontanezen memo: Wells Army Records, August 28 and September 20, 1919.

11. Pulaski Courthouse: Association of Arkansas Counties, "About Central Arkansas-Pulaski County," Office of Congressman Vic Snyder, http://www.house.gov/snyder/about_central_ar/pulaski.htm.

12. Quartermaster Corps: Quartermaster Museum, "The Quartermaster Remount Service," Army Quartermaster Foundation, http://www.qmfound.com/remount.htm.

13. Army Reorganization Act: Feller and Cox, *Highlights*, June 4, 1920.

14. Nineteenth Amendment ratification: Monroe, *Nineteenth Amendment,* 73-77; Wheeler, *One Woman, One Vote,* 333-36, 345.

15. Camp Lewis history: GlobalSecurity.org, "Army Forts and Camps-Fort Lewis," GlobalSecurity.org, http://www.globalsecurity.org/military/facility/fort-lewis.htm.

16. Vancouver trip: Wells Army Records, August 12, 1922.

17. Medical Examiner: Ibid., September 13, 1922.

18. George D. Wells Army discharge: Ibid., September 14, 1922.

Chapter Nine

1. "Martha Rose is so lively …": "Anderson Letters," January 14, 1924; September 25, 1924.

2. Signal Hill Oil: Paleontological Research Institution, "The Story of Oil in California-Signal Hill," Paleontological Research Institution, http://www.priweb.org/ed/pgws/history/signal_hill/signal_hill.html.

3. Ross Field: Richard DesChenes, "The Army Balloon School, Ross Field," The California State Military Museum, http://www.militarymuseum.org/BalloonSch.html.

4. Old Soldiers' Home: Veterans Park Conservancy, "Who We Are, What We Do, The Fields of Glory." Veterans Park Conservancy, http://www.veteranspark conservancy.org/.

5. Bell, CA: City of Bell, "Historical Background," City of Bell, http://www.gate waycog.org/bell/history.html.

6. Tribute to Fredrick Anderson: Fredrick Anderson Obituary, *Red Wing (MN) Republican Daily,*" March 8, 1932.

7. Tribute to Ellen Anderson: Ibid., April 9, 1936.

8. Vernon, CA: City of Vernon, "History," City of Vernon, http://www.cityof vernon.org/about_cov/history.htm.

9. Armistice Day at Los Angeles Coliseum: Los Angeles Times Archives, "Thousands Take Part in Armistice Services at Coliseum," November 11, 1924; "War Heroes Honored by Armistice Day Fete," November 12, 1925; "City Honors Heroes," November 11, 1927, accessed at Los Angeles Public Library database.

10. Veteran Affairs property: Veterans Park Conservancy, "Who We Are, What We Do, The Fields of Glory."

11. Army Nurse Corps GI Bill and equal rank: Feller and Cox, *Highlights*, September 1945, April 1947; Venzon, *United States*, 716.

12. Army Nurse Corps news: Feller and Cox, *Highlights*, July, 1950; February, and April, 1966.

13. Veterans Affairs property: Los Angeles National Cemetery, "General Information," "Historical Information," Los Angeles National Cemetery, http://www.cem.va.gov/CEM/cems/nchp/losangeles.asp.; Veterans Park Conservancy, "Who We Are, What We Do, The Fields of Glory"; United States Department of Veteran Affairs, "VA Greater Los Angeles Healthcare System (GLA)," Department of Veterans Affairs, http://www1.va.gov/directory/guide/facility.asp?ID=78.

Bibliography

Adams, Simon. *Eyewitness Books: World War I.* New York: Dorling Kindersley, 2001.

Bayne-Jones, Stanhope, MD. *The Evolution of Preventive Medicine in the United States Army, 1607-1939.* Washington, DC: GPO, 1968. Available online at http://history.amedd.army .mil/booksdocs/misc/evprev/.

Creel, George. *How We Advertised America.* New York: Harper & Brothers, 1920.

Feller, Carolyn M., Lt. Col., AN, USAR, and Maj. Debora R. Cox, AN, eds. *Highlights in the History of the Army Nurse Corps.* Washington, DC: U.S. Army Center of Military History, 2001. Available online at http://www.army.mil/cmh/ books/anc-highlights/highlights.htm.

Ford, Joseph H., Col., M.C. *The Medical Department of the United States Army in the World War.* Vol. 2, *Administration American Expeditionary Forces.* Washington, DC: GPO, 1927. Available online at http://history.amedd.army.mil/booksdocs/ wwi/adminamerexp/default.htm.

Ford, Joseph H., Col., M.C., Col. Charles Lynch, M.C., and Lt. Col. Frank W. Weed, M.C., *The Medical Department of the United States Army in the World War.* Vol. 8, *Field Operations.* Washington, DC: GPO, 1925. Available online at http:// history.amedd.army.mil/booksdocs/wwi/fieldoperations/ default.htm.

Ford, Nancy Gentile. *Americans All! Foreign-born Soldiers in World War I.* College Station: Texas A&M University Press, 2001.

Gavin, Lettie. *American Women in World War I: They Also Served.* Niwot: University Press of Colorado, 1997.

Grolier Library of World War I, The. 8 vols. Danbury, CT: Grolier Educational, 1997.

Hallas, James H., ed. *Doughboy War: The American Expeditionary Force in World War I.* Boulder, CO: Lynne Rienner Publishers, 2000.

History of World War I. 3 vols. New York: Marshall Cavendish, 2002.

Mankiller, Wilma, Gwendolyn Mink, Marysa Navarro, Barbara Smith, and Gloria Steinem, eds. *The Reader's Companion to U.S. Women's History*. New York: Houghton Mifflin, 1998.

Monroe, Judy. *The Nineteenth Amendment: Women's Right to Vote*. Springfield, NJ: Enslow Publishers, 1998.

Rasmussen, C.A. *History of Red Wing*. Red Wing, MN: privately published, 1933.

Sarnecky, Mary T., Col. USA (Ret.) *A History of the U.S. Army Nurse Corps*. Philadelphia: University of Pennsylvania Press, 1999.

Schneider, Dorothy and Carl J. Schneider. *Into the Breach: American Women Overseas in World War I*. New York: Viking Penguin, 1991.

Thatcher, Virginia S. *History of Anesthesia With Emphasis on the Nurse Specialist*. Philadelphia: J. B. Lippincott, 1953.

Venzon, Anne Cipriano, ed. *The United States in the First World War, An Encyclopedia*. New York: Garland Publishing, 1995.

Wheeler, Marjorie Spruill, ed. *One Woman, One Vote: Rediscovering the Woman Suffrage Movement*. Troutdale, OR: NewSage Press, 1995.

Young, Peter, Brig., ed. in chief. *The Marshall Cavendish Illustrated Encyclopedia of World War I*. 12 Vols. New York: Marshall Cavendish, 1984.

Electronic Material

American Association of Nurse Anesthetists. "AANA Overview." "History of Nurse Anesthesia Practice."American Association of Nurse Anesthetists. http://www.aana.com/aboutaana.aspx.

American Red Cross Museum. "American Red Cross Nursing." "World War I Accomplishments of the American Red Cross." American Red Cross. http://www.redcross.org/museum/history/.

Ancestry.com. "World War I Draft Registration Cards, 1917-1918." Ancestry.com. http://content.ancestry.com/iexec/?htx=List&dbid=6482&offerid=0:7858:0.

Arlington National Cemetery. "Samuel Davis Sturgis, Jr." Arlington National Cemetery. http://www.arlingtoncemetery.net/sturgisj.htm.

Association of Arkansas Counties. "About Central Arkansas-Pulaski County." Office of Congressman Vic Snyder. http://www.house.gov/snyder/about_central_ar/pulaski.htm.

Bryan, Jami L. "Fighting for Respect: African-American Soldiers in WW1." Army History Research. Army Historical Foundation. http://www.armyhistory.org/armyhistorical.aspx?pgID=868&id=103&exCompID=32.

Bunts, Alexander and George Crile, Jr. "The Founders." The Cleveland Clinic. http://www.clevelandclinic.org/act/Section1.pdf.

City of Bell, California. "Historical Background." City of Bell. http://www.gatewaycog.org/bell/history.html.

City of Vernon, California. "History." City of Vernon. http://www.cityofvernon.org/about_cov/history.htm.

DesChenes, Richard. "The Army Balloon School, Ross Field" The California State Military Museum. http://www.militarymuseum.org/BalloonSch.html.

Doughboy Center. *The Story of the American Expeditionary Forces.* The Great War Society. http://www.worldwar1.com/dbc.

FirstWorldWar.com. "Touring the Battlefields: the First Battlefield Tours." FirstWorldWar.com. http://www.firstworldwar.com/tours/firsttours.htm.

GlobalSecurity.org. "Army Forts and Camps – Fort Lewis." GlobalSecurity.org. http://www.globalsecurity.org/military/facility/fort-lewis.htm.

Knox, Dudley W., Capt. "American Naval Participation in the Great War (With Special Reference to the European Theater of Operations)." Washington, DC: Department of the Navy, Naval Historical Center, 2003. http://www.history.navy.mil/library/special/american_naval_part_great_war.htm.

Learning Centers at Ancestry.com. "Chart of World War I National Army Cantonments." Rootsweb.com. http://free pages.military.rootsweb.com/~worldwarone/WWI/Maps/chart.html.

Los Angeles National Cemetery. "General Information." "Historical Information." Los Angeles National Cemetery. http://www.cem.va.gov/CEM/cems/nchp/losangeles.asp.

Los Angeles Times Archives. "Thousands Take Part in Armistice Services at Coliseum," November 11, 1924; "War Heroes Honored by Armistice Day Fete," November 12, 1925; "City Honors War Heroes," November 11, 1927. Accessed at Los Angeles Public Library database.

Minnesota Historical Society. "Sea Wing Disaster." Minnesota Historical Society. http://www.mnhs.org/school/online/communities/milestones/milestones_sea_wing_disaster.htm.

The Ohio State University Department of History. "Clash of Cultures in the 1910s and 1920s - The New Woman." http://history.osu.edu/projects/Clash/NewWoman/newwomen-page1.htm (accessed May 4, 2006; site now discontinued). See http://history.osu.edu/.

Old State House Museum. "Arkansas Camp Has Major Role in the Great War." Old State House Museum. Search for Camp Pike at http://www.oldstatehouse.com/.

O'Shea, John S., MD. "Responding to Crisis: Franklin H. Martin, the ACS, and the Great War." *Bulletin of the American College of Surgeons*. Vol. 89, no. 6. The American College of Surgeons. http://www.facs.org/fellows_info/bulletin/2004/oshea0604.pdf.

Paleontological Research Institution. "The Story of Oil in California – Signal Hill." Paleontological Research Institution. http://www.priweb.org/ed/pgws/history/signal_hill/signal_hill.html.

Quartermaster Museum. "The Quartermaster Remount Service." Army Quartermaster Foundation. http://www.qmfound.com/remount.htm.

Taubenberger, Jeffery K., and David M. Morens. "1918 Influenza: the Mother of All Pandemics." Centers for Disease Control and Prevention. http://www.cdc.gov/ncidod/EID/vol12no01/05-0979.htm.

United States Army Center of Military History. "42nd Infantry Division History." Center of Military History. http://www.42id.army.mil/history/index.html.

United States Department of Defense. "DOD Principal Wars in Which the United States Participated, U.S. Military Personnel Serving and Casualties." Department of Defense. http://siadapp.dmdc.osd.mil/personnel/CASUALTY/WCPRINCIPAL.pdf.

United States Department of Veteran Affairs. "VA Greater Los Angeles Healthcare System (GLA)." Department of Veterans Affairs. http://www1.va.gov/directory/guide/facility.asp?ID=78.

United States National Archives and Records Administration. "World War I Selective Service System Draft Registration Cards." National Archives and Records Administration. http://www.archives.gov/genealogy/military/ww1/draft-registration/.

Veterans Park Conservancy. "Who We Are, What We Do, The Fields of Glory." Veterans Park Conservancy. http://www.veteransparkconservancy.org/.

Wilson, Woodrow. "War Message to Congress." April 2, 1917. Brigham Young University Library. http://www.lib.byu.edu/~rdh/wwi/1917/wilswarm.html.

Unpublished Materials

The following are from the Anderson Wells Memorabilia, a Private Collection.

Andersen, Andreas Fredrick. "Biography of the Andersens," 1927.

Anderson, Ellen Matilda. "Letters from Europe," 1906.

Anderson, Grace Matilda. "Grace Anderson Letters, 1917-1925."

United States Army Medical Corps Records of George Dillard Wells. War Department, Office of the Surgeon General. Washington, DC. 1917-1922.

United States Army Nurse Corps Records of Grace M. Anderson. War Department, Office of the Surgeon General. Washington, D.C. 1917-1919.

Other Sources

Goodhue County Historical Society, Red Wing, MN. Researched and accessed *History of Red Wing* and Anderson family obituaries from the Red Wing newspaper archives. *Red Wing (MN) Daily Republican*, 1918; *Red Wing (MN) Republican Daily*, 1932, 1936; *Red Wing (MN) Republican Eagle Daily*, 1959; *Red Wing (MN) Daily Republican Eagle*, 1965.

Greene County Archives & Records Center, Springfield, MO. Research of Webster County, MO, census records and Wells family burials at Shiloh Cemetery in Webster County, MO.

Museum of Ventura County. Patriotism and Persuasion: Posters of World War I. Ventura, CA. June 3 – August 28, 2005.

INDEX

adoption, 110

African-Americans, 16. *See also* blacks, Negroes.

American Ambulance Hospital (France), 34

American Expeditionary Forces (AEF), U.S. Army: AEF headquarters, 72; Ambulance Co., No. 111, Twenty-eighth Division dressing station, 54; Ambulance Co. No. 316, Seventy-ninth Division dressing station, 57; army and marines, 34; base hospital site selection, 49; battle injuries, 55-56; Belleau Wood, Battle of, 101, 146; casualty statistics, 56; Chateau-Thierry, Battle of, 50, 101-2, 148; demobilization, 87; embarkation, troops, 31, 40; Field Hospital No. 1, Second Division, 58; First Division first aid, 53; Forty-second Division triage, 59; Fourth Division field hospitals, 62; King George V message, 42-43; Marne, Second Battle of the, 47-48, 53, 148; Meuse-Argonne, Battle of, 53-54, 62, 146; Pontanezen, Camp, 45-46, 122, 124-25; return to U.S., 119-20; Spanish influenza, 62-63, 64; St. Mihiel, Battle of, 50, 105; train transport, 65; transport to Europe, 40-41; troopship activities, 42; wounded, Argonne Forest, 55

American Library Association, 19, 20

American Medical Association, 141

American new woman, 8-9

American Red Cross: base hospitals' formation, 34-36; contributions, public, 7; German refugees, 109; Germany, nurses, 111-12; membership, 7; posters, 7; recreation in France, 83-84; recruitment, nurses, 7-8; Red Cross mercy ship, 1; survival gear, xiii, 44; troop postcards, 43; uniforms, nurses, 33; Vichy Christmas, 85-86; volunteer workers, 7, 32; war prisoners, 84-85

Anderson, Arthur, xvii-xviii

Anderson, Clarence: anesthetist training, 21, 71; first letter, "over there," 43; grave of, 124; illness, death, 93-94; Mayo Clinic anesthetists, 22; Mayo Clinic physician, xviii; obituary, 94-95; volunteer, war service, 61, 96

Anderson, Ellen, xvii, 6, 141

Anderson, Fredrick, xvi, xvii, 6, 141

Anderson, Fredrick Edward, xviii

anesthesia administration, 21, 22, 69, 71-72, 80-81

anesthetist: Anderson, nurse anesthetist, xiv; anesthesia, 71; anesthesia departments, base hospitals, 71; anesthetist course, xviii, 35; anesthetist skills, 72; anesthetists, Walter Reed General Hospital, 71; army anesthetist program, 21, 71; chief anesthetist, 72, 77, 80-81; civilian anesthetists, 71; early army anesthetist, 22, 71; Mayo Clinic anesthetics course, 71; Mayo Clinic anesthetists, 22; teacher, anesthetists, 21

anti-German sentiment, 7

Arkansas: army discharge in, 125; attractive weather in, 28; Camp Pike site in, 12; marriage in, 126; move from, 129; nurses needed in, 28; recruits from, 11; troops' training in, 27

Army, U.S. *See* U.S. Army.

Army Medical Department, U.S. *See* U.S. Army Medical Department, American Expeditionary Forces.

Army-Navy Nurse Act, 144

Army Nurse Corps, U.S. *See* U.S. Army Nurse Corps.
Army Reorganization Act, 128

Baker, Elizabeth Leopold, 28, 29
Baker, Newton, D., 17
Baker, Robert S., 134
Base Hospital No. 17, AEF, army nurses: crisis expansion, 54-55; hospital history, 48; hospital photo, 48; lifestyle, 51-53, 60, 61, 64, 65; nurses' quarters, 49, 51, 52; nursing duty, 50, 54, 55, 56-57, 59-60; Spanish influenza patients, 61-64
Base Hospital No. 115, AEF, army nurses: chief nurse, 70, 78, 92; Christmas gift, 85-86; commanding officer, 78, 85; embarkation, xiii, 37, 41; group photo, 39; hospital closed, 99; hotel quarters, 69-70; Hotel Ruhl, 67, 68; King George V message, 42-43; leave, 86, 87-88, 90-91; lifestyle, 74, 76, 77-78, 84; mobilization, 31, 32, 33, 37; nurse anesthetist, xiv, xviii, 21-22, 35, 69, 71-72, 77, 80-81; nurses' song, xiii, 38; nursing duty, 69, 70-71, 77, 80, 93; overseas duty, motivation, xiii, xiv; recreation, events, 83-84; submarine trip, 45; survival gear, xiii, 44; team spirit, 70; temporary orders, 45-46; train travel, 75; troop postcard, 43; troopship voyage, 41, 42, 44; unit organized, 36
base hospitals, AEF: Base No. 1, 67, 73, 96, 122; Base No. 4, 35; Base No. 8, 41; Base No. 9, 48-49; Base No. 12, 41; Base No. 13, 49; Base No. 18, 36, 48; Base No. 19, 67, 96; Base No. 26, 35; Base No. 45, 49; Base No. 76, 67, 73, 79, 99; Base No. 93, 49; Base No. 109, 67-68, 70, 109
Bell, Bessie S., 9
Bell, Calif., 134-35, 136-40, passim, 141, 142
Belleau Wood, Battle of, 101, 146
Bellevue Hospital, 36, 67, 122, 124
Bellini, Giovanni, 85
blacks, 16-17
British Expeditionary Forces, 36

Caduceus, The, 84, 97
California: allure of, 132; army discharge in, 131; art galleries in, 142; cold winter in, 138; glowing reports of, 133; household moves in, xvi; medical examiner in, 131; physician, resident of, 144; Signal Hill in, 134; summer vacation in, 143; veterans in, 131
Camp Pike, U.S. Army: activities, camp, 19-20; army training, 11, 18, 27; athletic program, 28-29; Auxiliary Remount Depot, 127-28; construction, camp, 12-13; demographics, soldiers, 17-18; epidemics, camps, 16; immigrant soldiers, 17-18; name origin, camp, 11; racial prejudice, 16-17; site selection, 12; soldiers, U.S. camps, 28
Camp Pike, U.S. Army nurses: group photos, 25, 26, 29; hospital duty, 14, 16, 26; insurance policies, 23; lifestyle, 14, 16, 28; nurse anesthetists, 21-22; special events, 26, 27, 28, 29
cantonments, U.S. Army, 11, 12, 13, 16-18, 19-20, 28-29
Chateau-Thierry, Battle of, 50, 101-2, 148
Christy, Howard Chandler, 4, 5
Civil War, U.S., xvii, 21, 134

Wells Industrial Emergency Hospital, 141, 143, 144
Wells, Martha Rose, 125-26, 127, 128, 129, 135-36, 137-44 passim
Wells, Mollie, 127, 129, 143
Western Reserve University, 34
White House, the, 9, 76
Wilson, Woodrow, 2, 5, 9, 120, 122, 128
World War I: Allies, 1, 2, 32, 40, 47, 51; armed forces mobilization, 5; armistice
    celebrations, 70, 75, 76; Belleau Wood, Battle of, 101, 146; Central powers, 1;
    Chateau-Thierry, Battle of, 50, 101-2, 148; convoy system, 40; *Lusitania* attack, 2;
    Marne, Second Battle of the, 47-48, 53, 148; Meuse-Argonne, Battle of, 53-54, 62,
    146; military draft, 2, 4-5, 17; neutrality, U.S. policy, 1; Pershing, John J., 9, 115-
    16, 117; Reims war ruins, 103; Selective Service Act, 2; St. Mihiel, Battle of, 50,
    105; U-boat attacks, 2; unrestricted submarine campaign, 2, 38, 40; U.S.
    demobilization, 87; U.S. entry in war, 2-3, 4; Verdun war ruins, 104; Zimmermann
    Telegram, 2
World War II, 143-44

YMCA, 18, 19
YWCA, 19, 20

Zimmermann Telegram, 2